Somatic Exercises and Practices for Beginners:

Reset your Nervous System

Promote Emotional Awareness and Resilience

Clear Stagnant Energy from your Body

Improve Balance, Flexibility, and Posture

Lose Weight and Tone

Index

Introduction

$\mathcal{E}$very step we take in life is a chance to reconnect with our bodies and minds, yet so many of us walk through our days disconnected from the sensations that animate our existence. The power of somatic exercises — an intricate dance of movement, breath, and awareness — is often underestimated in its potential to transform lives. This book is born from my own journey, a path that led me from chronic discomfort and emotional turbulence to a place of greater peace and vitality through the practices I share here.

I am a certified Body Talk practitioner, with years dedicated to exploring and integrating various healing modalities. My passion for holistic health is not just professional; it is deeply personal. I have witnessed firsthand how somatic practices can liberate us from the shackles of pain and emotional instability. This book is an embodiment of my commitment to support women, whether they are yoga enthusiasts or those who feel disconnected from such practices due to being overweight, experiencing chronic pain, or carrying the heavy burdens of trauma.

Somatic exercises are a gateway to better understanding and nurturing our bodies. They are not just exercises; they are a form of communication with our deepest selves. Through movements that reset our nervous systems, promote emotional awareness, and clear stagnant energy, these practices encourage a harmonious dialogue between mind and body. Incorporating elements like Breathwork, Tapping, Vagus Nerve Stimulation, and Grounding, this book offers more than just physical postures; it offers pathways to resilience and joy.

The purpose of this book is clear: to provide a gentle yet effective guide for those new to somatic exercises as well as enriching insights for those at an intermediate level. You will find detailed instructions, helpful illustrations, and insights into the emotional and physical benefits of each practice. This is not just a manual; it's a companion in your journey towards a healthier, more balanced life.

Structured to be both informative and practical, this guide begins with foundational theories before moving into a diverse array of exercises that you can integrate into your daily routine. From spine stretches to mindful walking, each chapter builds on the last, crafting a holistic approach to health that suits a wide range of needs and fitness levels.

What sets this book apart is its commitment to inclusivity and practicality. It combines rigorous exercise guides with advice on nutrition and mindfulness, supplemented by motivational tips. High-quality illustrations accompany each exercise, making the practices accessible to all, regardless of prior knowledge or experience.

To you, the reader, I know the road to healing can seem daunting. You may feel hindered by physical discomfort or emotional scars. Yet, here is a tool that promises not just relief but transformation. I invite you to engage with this book not just as a reader, but as an active participant in your own journey of healing and self-discovery.

Let's begin this transformative journey together, one breath, one stretch, one mindful moment at a time.

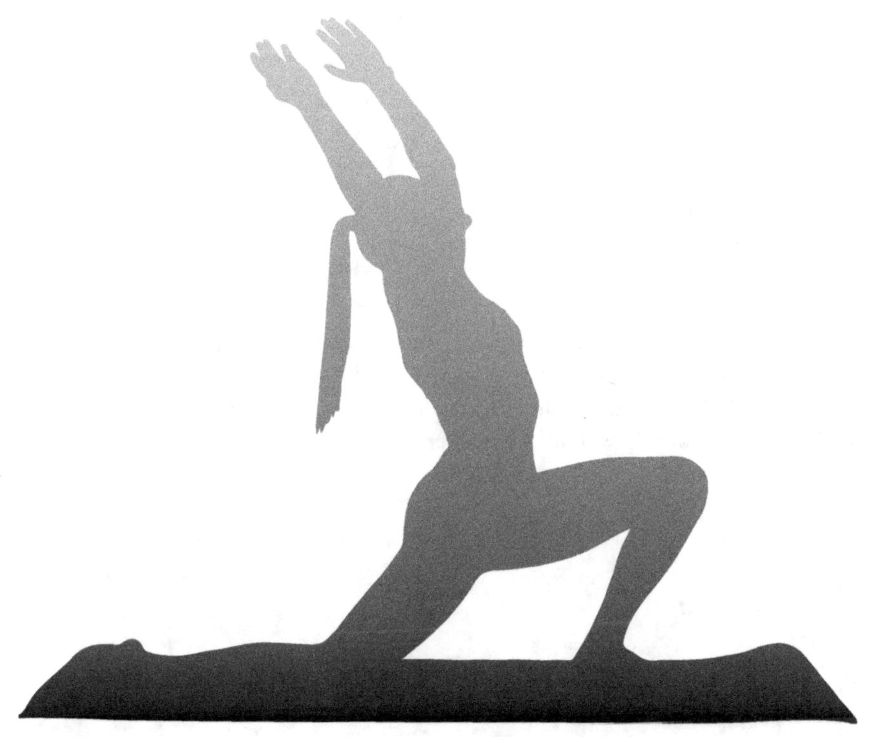

Chapter 1: *Introduction to Somatics*

Have you ever felt as if your body is speaking, perhaps whispering hints or shouting demands, and yet somehow the message gets lost in the noise of daily life? Somatics is about tuning into that dialogue, engaging with the subtle and not-so-subtle cues that our bodies give us. It's a practice that doesn't just change bodies; it transforms lives by fostering a deep, intrinsic connection between the mind and the physical self. This first chapter is your gateway into understanding how somatic exercises work their magic, starting with the very core of our being: the nervous system.

As we explore the intricate dance between our physical actions and neurological responses, you'll discover how somatic practices offer more than just physical benefits—they are a key to unlocking emotional resilience and a deeper sense of well-being. Whether you're dealing with the stressors of daily life, managing chronic pain, or seeking to improve your overall health, the insights and exercises shared here are designed to bring you back into balance, into a state of harmony where your body and mind are aligned and attuned.

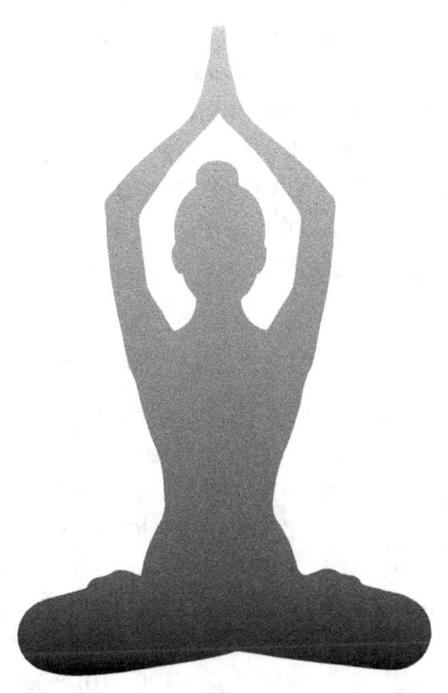

1.1 The Science Behind Somatics: Resetting the Nervous System

Understanding the Nervous System

Our nervous system is the command center for the body, directing traffic, sending signals, and making sure messages get where they need to go for our survival and well-being. It's helpful to think of it as a complex network, much like a busy city's traffic system, controlling everything from quick, reflexive responses to calculated movements. Somatic exercises serve as a type of traffic control, helping to manage the flow and ensuring that the nervous system responds appropriately to stimuli. By practicing somatic exercises, you're essentially teaching your body new, healthier ways to respond to the stresses and strains of life. Somatic Yoga is named after the Somatic Nervous system. Sometimes, these nerves have forgotten or lost the ability to control muscles in certain parts of our bodies; leading to stiffness and chronic pain. Somatic Yoga exercises can help relax these muscles by releasing tension and re-establishing the brain-to-muscle connection.

Fight or Flight vs. Rest and Digest

You've likely heard of the "fight or flight" response, our body's ancient alarm system that prepares us to either fight or flee when faced with danger. This response is controlled by the sympathetic nervous system. On the flip side, there's the "rest and digest" system, managed by the parasympathetic nervous system, which takes over when the body is at rest. It's responsible for processes that occur when the body is relaxed, such as digestion and healing. Somatic exercises activate this parasympathetic response, which is crucial for stress relief and healing. Through targeted movements and mindful practices, somatic exercises encourage the body to shift from high alert to a state of calm and relaxation, promoting a balance often lost in our hectic lifestyles.

Neuroplasticity and Somatics

One of the most exciting aspects of somatic exercises is their ability to mold and shape our brain's responses, thanks to neuroplasticity. This term refers to the brain's ability to reorganize itself by forming new neural connections throughout life. Somatic practices leverage this capability by creating new, healthier patterns of response in our nervous system. Regular practice can help reroute old patterns of the fight or flight response, making calm and relaxation more automatic responses to stressors. This reshaping of the brain's reactions can have profound implications for healing from trauma and managing chronic stress.

Benefits of a Balanced Nervous System

A well-balanced nervous system isn't just about feeling less stressed. It's about unlocking the body's inherent ability to heal and maintain equilibrium. Benefits include improved sleep quality, fewer feelings of anxiety, better management of chronic pain, and enhanced emotional resilience. These changes can create a positive feedback loop: a calmer nervous system leads to better sleep and less pain, which in turn leads to more effective management of stress and anxiety, reinforcing the calm state of relaxation.

In this chapter, you've begun to peel back the layers of how somatic exercises influence and interact with our nervous system. As you continue to explore and apply these practices, you're not just performing exercises; you're engaging in a form of deep listening and communication with your body, a dialogue that can lead to profound healing and transformation.

1.2 Breathing Techniques for Emotional Balance and Stress Relief

The simple act of breathing, something we often do without a second thought, holds incredible power over our physical and emotional states. It's fascinating, isn't it? How the way we breathe, can change the way we feel? By adjusting our breath, we can directly influence our body's stress response, calming our minds and soothing our nervous systems. This section explores the profound impact that breathwork can have on achieving emotional stability and how you can harness this power to enhance your daily life and deepen your somatic practice.

Breathing is intimately connected to our emotions. Consider how your breathing changes when you're anxious or scared—short, shallow breaths that seem to heighten your alertness and tension. Conversely, when relaxed, your breath becomes deeper and more rhythmic, naturally guiding you to a calmer state. This isn't just a reflex; it's a tool we can consciously utilize to manage our emotions. By learning and practicing specific breathing techniques, you can not only counteract daily stress but also cultivate a profound sense of emotional balance. These techniques, grounded in centuries of traditional practices, have been validated by contemporary research which shows that controlled breathing can reduce cortisol levels—the stress hormone—and enhance the production of endorphins, the body's natural painkillers and mood elevators.

Let's explore some basic yet powerful breathing exercises. A fundamental technique is diaphragmatic breathing, or belly breathing, which involves breathing deeply into the belly rather than the chest. This type of breathing stimulates the vagus nerve, playing a crucial role in initiating a relaxation response throughout the body. To practice, simply sit comfortably or lie down, place one hand on your abdomen, and breathe in slowly through your nose, feeling your belly rise. Then breathe out through your mouth, letting your belly fall. This technique is particularly effective in moments of acute stress, as it helps shift the body's response away from fight or flight and toward rest and digest.

Integrating these breathing techniques into your everyday life can be surprisingly simple, yet it requires a mindful commitment. One effective way to ensure you are practicing regularly is to link your breathing exercises to daily activities. For instance, practice ten deep breaths before each meal. It's a practical way to reduce stress and can also aid in digestive processes, making it a dual-purpose exercise. Another tip is to use breathwork as a transitional tool. For example, if you transition from a hectic workday to personal time, use five minutes of focused breathing to help delineate and mentally separate these parts of your day. This not only helps in managing stress but also improves your presence and engagement in your activities following the exercise.

Understanding why these techniques are vital for advancing in somatic exercises opens up a deeper layer of practice. In somatic exercises, breathwork is not just a preliminary warm-up but integral to the practice itself. Each breath can be synchronized with movements to enhance the efficacy of the exercise, deepen the experience, and increase the release of bodily tensions. Mastering breathing not only improves the execution of somatic movements but also enhances the connection between your mind and body, making each session more impactful.

By now, it's clear that breathwork is not merely a supplementary exercise but a foundational practice for emotional and physical health. As you continue to explore these techniques, you may find yourself becoming more attuned to the nuances of your body's responses. This awareness is a powerful tool—think of it as learning a new language, the language of your own body, which will support you not just in somatic practices but in every aspect of life.

1.3 Tapping into Wellness: An Introduction to EFT and Quantum Tapping

Emotional Freedom Technique, or EFT as it is more commonly known, and Quantum Tapping might sound like something out of a modern self-help guide, but it's rooted in ancient healing practices. EFT involves tapping on specific points on the body, similar to acupressure, to release emotional blockages, thereby improving emotional health. This technique, often referred to as 'tapping', has been a transformative tool for many, providing relief from emotional distress, anxiety, and more. It's a simple yet profound way to reconnect with your body while calming the mind.

Many forms of Quantum Tapping provide energy healing and emotional release, using tapping techniques to create a powerful shift in the mind-body matrix. One form of Quantum Tapping involves simultaneously tapping the head and heart, and then the head and gut. This can be very effective in stressful situations; to relieve feelings of anxiety and to restore balance to your body.

The science behind tapping is as fascinating as the practice itself. Each tapping point is located on meridians used in traditional Chinese medicine, pathways within the body along which vital energy flows. When you tap these points with your fingertips, you're essentially sending signals to the brain to calm the fight or flight response, transitioning to a state of relaxation. This response can be attributed to the reduction in cortisol (a stress hormone) levels and the increase in endorphins, the body's natural painkillers and mood enhancers. This biochemical shift in the body can dramatically reduce or even eliminate emotional distress.

For those new to EFT, here's a beginner-friendly guide to get you started: First, identify the issue you want to focus on, whether it's anxiety, fear, or any distressing emotion. Acknowledge this issue and accept yourself despite it. Begin by tapping on the karate chop point (the outer edge of your hand) while stating your issue aloud, followed by an affirmation of self-acceptance. For example, you might say, "Even though I feel anxious about my presentation, I deeply and completely accept myself." Next, tap about 7 times on each of the following points in sequence: the eyebrow, side of the eye, under the eye, under the nose, the chin, the beginning of the collarbone, and under the arm. While tapping, maintain a focus on your emotion and observe any shift in your feelings.

Incorporating EFT into somatic practices offers a holistic approach to wellness by addressing not just the physical but also the emotional layers of our being. While somatic exercises often focus on physical sensations and movements, EFT directly targets emotional barriers that might be hindering physical progress. For example, if chronic pain is linked to emotional stress, tapping can alleviate some of this emotional weight, potentially reducing the physical symptoms as well. In this way, EFT complements somatic exercises, creating a more comprehensive approach to health that acknowledges the intricate connection between the body and the mind.

EFT is particularly empowering because it places emotional regulation tools directly into your hands—quite literally. It encourages a deep engagement with your emotional landscape, promoting a transformative self-awareness. This practice can be done anywhere and requires only a few minutes, making it an excellent technique for those who lead busy lives but still want to maintain a focus on personal wellness. As you continue to use EFT along with other somatic practices, you might find greater ease in navigating the challenges that come your way, armed with tools that support not just your body but your emotional and mental landscapes as well.

1.4 The Role of the Vagus Nerve in Emotional Regulation

Imagine the vagus nerve as a serene river flowing through your body, touching various organs with gentle whispers of calm and reassurance. This nerve is not just any river, though; it is the longest cranial nerve in your body, connecting your brain to many important organs involved in digestion, heart rate, and respiratory rate. Its role in the parasympathetic nervous system is to manage your body's relaxation phases—those peaceful moments when you are at rest. Understanding the vagus nerve is akin to discovering a hidden control panel in your body that can help manage stress and usher in an immense sense of calm.

The vagus nerve acts like a bi-directional superhighway, carrying an array of signals from the brain to the body and vice versa. When it's functioning optimally, it tells your body that it's time to relax, encouraging your heart rate to slow down and your digestion to engage fully—essentially promoting a "rest and digest" state. This nerve also has a significant impact on how you handle emotional stress. When activated, it helps to quell the anxiety-inducing messages that might be ping-ponging around your nervous system. This activation not only helps in immediate stress relief but also aids in building a resilience that can transform your response to stress over time.

Stimulating the vagus nerve is remarkably simple and can be incorporated into various daily activities to promote relaxation and emotional well-being. Somatic exercises, such as deep and slow abdominal breathing, are particularly effective. When you engage in deep breathing, you indirectly massage the vagus nerve which runs through your diaphragm, sending a signal to your body to shift into a state of calm. Another effective method is singing or chanting, which involves the muscles in the back of the throat—another area connected to the vagus nerve. Even gargling regularly or engaging in light, mindful humming can activate this pivotal nerve.

Building resilience through regular vagus nerve stimulation can be a game changer in managing emotional health. Think of resilience as an emotional muscle that, when strengthened, can help you bounce back quicker from life's ups and downs. You're essentially training this muscle by regularly practicing exercises that stimulate the vagus nerve. You teach your body how to switch more efficiently from a state of stress to a state of relaxation, which, over time, enhances your overall emotional health, making you less reactive to stress and more capable of handling anxiety and depression.

Here are a few practical exercises you can incorporate into your daily routine to stimulate your vagus nerve:

1. **Diaphragmatic Breathing**: Sit or lie comfortably, placing one hand on your belly. Slowly inhale through your nose, allowing your belly to rise, then exhale gently either through your nose or mouth, letting your belly fall. Aim for 6 to 8 breaths per minute, focusing on long, deep breaths.

2. **Singing or Chanting**: Integrate singing into your daily life, whether it's singing along to your favorite song on the radio or chanting a mantra during meditation. The act of singing works the muscles in the back of your throat to stimulate the vagus nerve.

3. **Gargling**: A simple practice you can do every morning or night. After brushing your teeth, take a sip of water, tilt your head back, and gargle vigorously for a few seconds. Repeat a few times to activate the vagus nerve at the back of the throat.

Incorporating these practices doesn't require drastic changes to your lifestyle, yet they can lead to profound improvements in how you feel emotionally and physically. As with any new habit, the key is consistency. The more regularly you engage in vagus nerve stimulation exercises, the more you'll notice improvements in your stress levels and emotional well-being.

1.5 Grounding Exercises for Energy and Focus

Imagine standing barefoot on a cool patch of earth, feeling a soft breeze and the gentle warmth of the sun—this simple act is often overlooked, yet it's profoundly connected to our well-being. Grounding, sometimes referred to as earthing, involves direct skin contact with the surface of the Earth, such as bare feet or hands touching the soil, grass, or sand. The concept, deeply embedded in some indigenous cultures and holistic health practices, is based on the idea that the Earth's natural charge can help stabilize the body's basic biological rhythms and reduce inflammation and pain.

Grounding is not just about physical connection with the earth; it's about anchoring yourself in the present moment and reconnecting with your environment, which can often feel lost in the hustle of modern life. This reconnection is crucial for those of us dealing with daily stresses, chronic pain, or emotional upheavals. Incorporating grounding techniques into your life can be a simple, yet powerful way to enhance focus, stabilize your energy, and cultivate a serene mind.

For beginners, grounding can be as simple as walking barefoot. If you're able to, find a safe, clean patch of grass or sand and spend a few minutes walking or standing barefoot. Feel each touch between your feet and the earth. Notice the temperature, the textures, and any sensations that arise in your body. This practice helps reduce the stress hormone cortisol, which when elevated, can disrupt many body processes. Another technique involves lying on the ground - use a park or your backyard on a pleasant day to lie down and let your body be supported by the earth. Close your eyes, breathe deeply, and feel the connection to the ground beneath you. Focus on the points of contact between your body and the earth and imagine tension draining away from your body and into the earth.

Integrating grounding into your daily routine can be creatively simple and highly effective. Those who spend a lot of time indoors should consider getting a grounding mat. These mats mimic the earth's electric potential and can be used while sitting or sleeping. Place one under your desk or in your relaxation area. Make a habit of using it for a few minutes each day—perhaps during a morning meditation, while reading a book, or even while working at your desk. For those who can step outside, try starting your morning by standing or walking barefoot outside for a few minutes. This practice not only wakes up your senses but also sets a calm, grounded tone for the day.

The benefits of regular grounding practice are not just anecdotal; they are supported by emerging scientific research suggesting that grounding can improve sleep, reduce chronic pain, and decrease stress. Over time, these benefits contribute to greater emotional stability and physical health. Imagine grounding as a stabilizing force, like roots that keep a tree steady in changing weather. It enhances your life's quality by increasing your presence in the now, improving your focus, and stabilizing your internal environment regardless of the external chaos.

As we move through our days, often rushed and disconnected, grounding offers a way to slow down and sync up with the world around us. It reminds us that we are not just inhabitants of this earth but a part of it. By regularly practicing grounding techniques, you're not just touching the earth; you're tapping into a source of natural healing and stability, which in turn nurtures your overall well-being and prepares you to handle the complexities of life with renewed energy and focus. As you continue to explore and integrate these practices, notice the subtle yet profound ways in which they enhance your connection to your body, to the earth, and to the present moment.

1.6 Body Scanning for Awareness and Pain Relief

Imagine for a moment that you could communicate with your body, not through words but through a gentle and attentive scan, from the crown of your head down to the tips of your toes. This is the essence of body scanning, a mindfulness practice that invites you to tune into your body, part by part, to discover how each area feels. It's akin to a radiologist using an MRI machine to look inside the body, except in this practice, your mind is the scanner, and the body parts are the subjects being observed. This method is not just about identifying discomfort or tension; it's about cultivating a deeper awareness of your physical self, which can lead to profound healing and pain relief.

Body scanning operates on a simple yet powerful premise: that mindful attention directed towards the body can alter one's experience of pain and stress. When you perform a body scan, you lie down, close your eyes, and focus your attention systematically on each part of your body. You might start at your feet, noticing any sensations, warmth, tingling, or perhaps nothing at all. You then mentally note these sensations and gently move your focus up to the ankles, calves, knees, and so forth, up through the entire body. The key here is observation without judgment or the need to change anything. This practice can unearth areas of tension and discomfort that you were previously unaware of, simply because so much of our daily lives is spent disconnected from our physical selves.

The technique is particularly effective in reducing stress and promoting relaxation. As you scan your body, your nervous system begins to shift from a state of alertness to one of calm. This happens because focusing your attention in a non-reactive way sends a signal to your brain that there is no immediate threat in the environment, allowing your body to initiate its relaxation responses. This can be especially beneficial if you're dealing with chronic pain or recovering from trauma, as these conditions can keep your body in a heightened state of stress. By regularly practicing body scanning, you create a safe space for your body to relax and start the healing process.

Integrating body scans into your somatic practice enhances the benefits of other exercises by fostering greater bodily awareness. For instance, if during a body scan, you notice tension in your shoulders, you can then use targeted somatic exercises to release this tension. Over time, this heightened awareness can lead to more intuitive movements and a deeper understanding of what your body needs to heal and thrive. It also facilitates a deeper emotional release because, as you become more attuned to the physical sensations within your body, you also become more aware of the emotions associated with these sensations. This awareness can be transformative, allowing you to process and release emotions that may have been stored in the body for years.

To begin incorporating body scans into your routine, try scheduling a regular time each day for this practice. Early morning or right before bed are ideal times as they are typically quieter moments of the day. Start with just five minutes, focusing on breathing deeply and scanning through each body part slowly. As you become more comfortable with the practice, you can extend the duration, allowing more time to really tune in to each area of your body. Remember, the goal is not to rush or to fix anything but to observe and connect with your body.

Through regular practice, body scanning can become a cornerstone of your self-care routine, offering a simple yet profound way to reduce stress, manage pain, and connect more deeply with yourself. It teaches patience and compassionate attention, reminding us that healing is not always about doing more or being more but about being present and attentive to our current experience. This mindful presence, cultivated through body scanning, is a powerful tool in the journey toward holistic health and well-being. As you continue to engage with this practice, you may find that the greatest communication does not come through words but through the silent language of attentive presence.

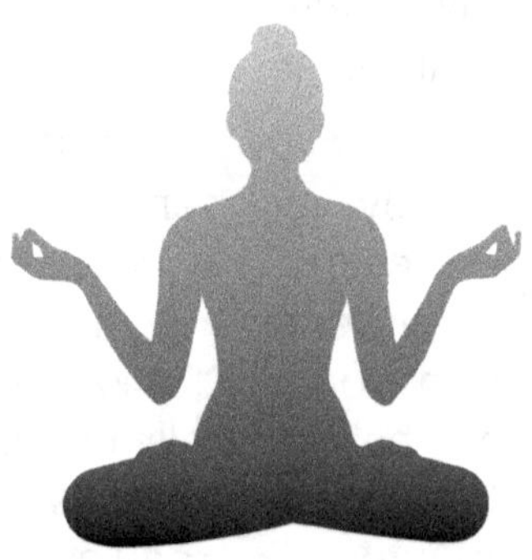

Chapter 2: Beginner's Guide to Key Somatic Exercises

Imagine your spine as the central highway of your body, a crucial conduit through which the essential communications of your nervous system travel. Its health and alignment influence everything from your posture to your well-being, impacting how you feel both physically and emotionally every day. This chapter is dedicated to exploring the foundational element of spinal health through somatic exercises, aiming to enhance your flexibility, improve your posture, and enrich your overall quality of life. Let's gently unfold the layers of spinal care, ensuring that each movement and stretch brings you closer to a state of balance and health.

2.1 Spine Stretches for Flexibility and Posture Improvement

Importance of Spinal Health

Your spine's health is paramount; it is the pillar that supports your movements, the protector of your central nervous system, and the core from which your body's balance and alignment are regulated. Maintaining spinal health is not just about avoiding discomfort; it's about enhancing your body's overall functionality and vitality. Somatic exercises designed for spinal health focus on improving flexibility and posture, which can alleviate common issues such as back pain and muscular tension, often exacerbated by our modern lifestyles that involve prolonged sitting and limited physical activity. By incorporating simple spine stretches into your daily routine, you can maintain the integrity of your spine and enhance your body's overall resilience and performance.

Simple Spine Stretching Exercises

Let's explore some beginner-friendly spine stretches that you can easily do at home. These exercises are designed to be gentle yet effective, catering to anyone, regardless of their fitness level or experience with somatic practices. *One fundamental stretch is the Cat-Cow Stretch, which involves positioning yourself on your hands and knees and gently alternating between arching your back towards the ceiling and dipping it towards the floor. This*

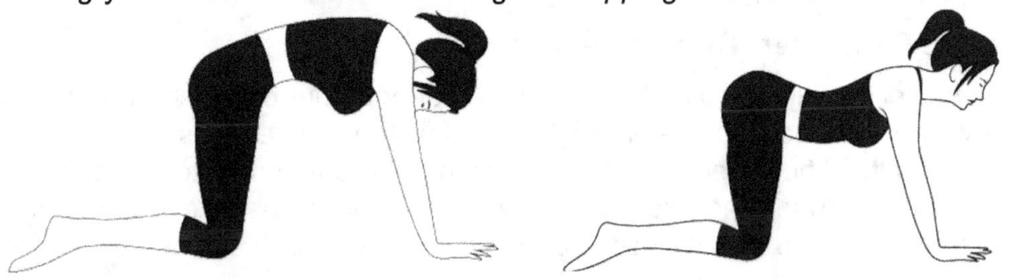

movement promotes spinal flexibility and can be particularly soothing for stiff back muscles. Another beneficial stretch is the spinal twist. *Sitting on the floor with your legs extended, bend one knee and place the opposite elbow on the outside of the bent knee, gently twisting your torso and looking over your shoulder.* This stretch not loosens the muscles around the spine but also helps detoxify your internal organs through the gentle squeezing action.

Integrating Spine Stretches into Daily Life

Incorporating spine stretches into your daily life can be straightforward and highly beneficial. Consider setting aside a specific time each day for your stretching routine, perhaps in the morning to awaken your body or in the evening to unwind after a day's activities. You can also integrate these stretches into your work breaks, especially if you spend long hours at a desk. Stretching not only breaks the monotony of prolonged sitting but also invigorates your spine, keeping it flexible and active. Another practical tip is to pair your stretching with daily habits, such as watching TV or listening to a podcast. This pairing makes the practice feel less like a chore and more like a natural part of your routine.

Safety Tips for Spine Stretching

While spine stretching is generally safe, proper technique and awareness are crucial to prevent injury and ensure the practice is beneficial. Always listen to your body and avoid pushing into pain. The goal of stretching is to feel a gentle pull, not pain. Start each stretch slowly, increasing the intensity only as far as your body comfortably allows. Pay attention to your breathing as well; ensure you are breathing steadily, as holding your breath can lead to unnecessary tension in your muscles. If you have existing back issues or health concerns, it's a wise idea to consult with a healthcare provider or a trained somatic exercise instructor who can guide you in adapting these stretches to your specific needs.

Gentle Reminder: Reflective Journaling

Consider keeping a reflective journal to deepen your connection with your body and enhance your awareness of how these exercises impact your spinal health. After each stretching session, take a few minutes to jot down what you felt during the exercises, any areas of tightness or ease, and how you feel afterward. This practice not only tracks your progress but also tunes you into the subtle languages of your body, fostering a deeper mind-body connection that is central to somatic practices.

In this section, we've navigated through the fundamentals of spinal health, from understanding its importance to integrating beneficial stretches into your daily routine. As you continue to explore these exercises, remember that each stretch is a step towards better health and greater harmony within your body. Embrace these movements with patience and mindfulness, and observe how they bring not only flexibility but also a profound sense of relief and alignment to your life.

2.2 Gentle Full Body Stretch: Awakening Your Senses

Imagine waking up each morning with a gentle stretching routine that not only eases you into the day but also invigorates your entire body, setting a tone of vitality and alertness. A full body stretch does more than just loosen up the muscles; it integrates your physical sensations with mental awareness, enhancing both your physical and emotional landscape. When you stretch every part of your body systematically, you're not only improving your flexibility but also increasing your blood flow, which can significantly boost your energy levels and overall vitality.

The beauty of a full body stretch lies in its simplicity and the profound impact it can have on your day-to-day life. Let's walk through a gentle routine that is suitable even for beginners and can be a cornerstone of your daily practice. Start by finding a quiet, comfortable space where you can stretch without interruptions. You might choose to have a yoga mat, but it's not essential. *Begin with your feet hip-width apart, standing tall, and take a deep, grounding breath. As you exhale, reach your arms towards the sky, lengthening your entire body. After a few seconds, gently swan dive over your legs, letting your head hang and your neck relax, feeling the stretch in your hamstrings and the release in your lower back.*

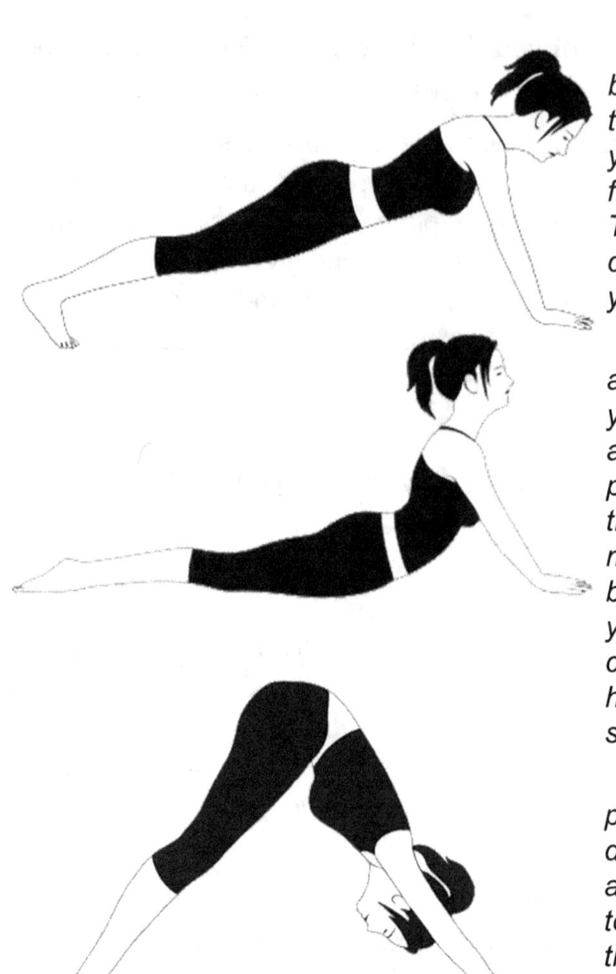

From this forward fold, step back into a plank position, taking a moment to ensure your body is in a straight line from your head to your heels. This not only engages your core but also strengthens your shoulders and arms.

After holding the plank for a few breaths, slowly lower your body to the ground and transition into a cobra pose by lifting your chest off the floor, using your back muscles to pull your torso back and up. This opens up your chest and shoulders, counteracting the forward hunch that comes from sitting at a desk.

To complete the cycle, push back into a downward dog, lifting your hips high and pressing your heels towards the ground, feeling the stretch in your calves and the decompression in your spine.

Integrating mindfulness into this routine amplifies its benefits. As you move through each stretch, pay close attention to the sensations in each part of your body. Notice where you feel tightness or ease, warmth or coolness. Mindfulness transforms stretching from a routine physical activity into a holistic practice that connects you deeply with your body's needs and capabilities. It teaches you to listen to your body's subtle cues, fostering a nurturing relationship where you respond to its needs with care and attentiveness.

Customizing your full body stretch routine is essential to make it truly beneficial for you. Each body is unique, with its own strengths and limitations, and acknowledging this is key to a successful somatic practice. If you find certain stretches too challenging, it's perfectly okay to modify them. For instance, if the full forward fold is uncomfortable, try bending your knees slightly or using a prop like a chair to support your hands. Always remember, the goal of stretching is not to achieve the perfect pose but to find the version of the pose that feels right for your body at that moment.

Encouraging yourself to maintain this practice daily can be transformative. Over time, as you continue to engage in full body stretches, you'll likely notice an improvement in your flexibility and a decrease in day-to-day stiffness. Your energy levels may increase, thanks to improved circulation and breathing that accompany regular stretching. Perhaps most importantly, you'll develop a more intimate understanding of your body's language, learning to hear what it needs and how best to provide for it. This dialogue with your body is a precious outcome of a consistent full body stretching routine, enriching both your physical health and your emotional well-being.

2.3 Elbow and Shoulder Stretches for Desk Workers

If you find yourself spending long hours at a desk, you're likely familiar with the stiffness and discomfort that can accumulate in your elbows and shoulders. These areas bear the brunt of repetitive movements and sustained postures, often leading to tension that not only feels uncomfortable but can also impact your overall mobility and health. With their gentle and focused approach, somatic exercises offer a pathway to relief and a strategy for prevention that can integrate seamlessly into your workday.

Let's talk about the common areas where desk workers often experience tension. The elbows and shoulders are pivotal points of movement that, when constrained by desk work, tend not to experience their full range of motion regularly. This limitation can lead to the buildup of tension and discomfort, manifesting as soreness, aching, or even sharp pain during movements. Recognizing these signs early is crucial in addressing them effectively through targeted somatic exercises. For instance, simple stretches that extend and rotate these joints can significantly alleviate discomfort and restore a sense of ease and fluidity to your movements.

Discovering effective stretches specifically designed for the elbows and shoulders can transform your work experience, turning a potentially painful desk job into a more comfortable and healthy endeavor. One beneficial stretch for the shoulders is the 'Pendulum Swing.' *Start by leaning slightly forward, supporting yourself with one hand on your desk, and let the other arm hang loosely. Gently swing this arm in small circles, gradually expanding the circles as your shoulder loosens.* This exercise encourages mobility without strain, lubricating the shoulder joint and easing tension. For the elbows, try the *'Wrist Walk' up a wall: face a wall, placing your palms against it at waist height, and slowly walking your fingers upwards, stretching the arms fully, then walking them back down. This not only stretches the elbow joints but also engages the muscles of the arms and shoulders, promoting blood flow and flexibility.*

Understanding how regular stretching can prevent repetitive strain injuries (RSIs) is fundamental, especially for desk workers. RSIs are injuries to the musculoskeletal and nervous systems that may be caused by repetitive tasks, forceful exertions, vibrations, mechanical compression, or sustained awkward positions. By incorporating regular elbow and shoulder stretches into your routine, you can maintain the elasticity of your muscles and tendons, and ensure that your joints remain lubricated and flexible. This proactive approach significantly reduces the risk of developing RSIs, making it an essential component of a healthy workspace routine.

One practical way to integrate these stretches into your day is by incorporating them into your regular work breaks. If you're like many people, taking breaks might consist of just stepping away from your desk or checking your phone. However, by using this time to stretch, you transform these pauses into opportunities for improving your health and well-being. Set a reminder every hour to take a short stretching break. Use this time to disconnect from work mentally and reconnect with your body physically. Even a few minutes spent stretching can help break the cycle of tension and prevent the accumulation of stress in your body.

As you incorporate these somatic exercises into your daily routine, you might find that they not only alleviate physical tension but also enhance your mental clarity and productivity. The act of stretching can provide a mental break, allowing you to return to your tasks refreshed and ready to engage. Over time, these small rituals of movement and mindfulness contribute to a more balanced work experience, where health and productivity go hand in hand, and taking care of your body is part of how you succeed every day.

2.4 The Superman Pose: Building Core Strength Gently

Imagine yourself as a superhero for a moment, not just in metaphor but in movement. The Superman pose, a simple yet powerful exercise, helps you embody strength and resilience, engaging your core in a way that supports your entire body's health. This pose is not about transforming into someone else; it's about uncovering the strength that resides within you, tapping into a core stability that enhances every other physical activity you engage in. Let's explore the Superman pose, understand its benefits, and learn how to safely integrate it into your daily routine to harness its full potential.

The core of your body, encompassing your abdominal muscles, lower back, hips, and pelvis, is the central link connecting your upper and lower body. The strength of this core is crucial for almost every movement you make and plays a pivotal role in your overall physical health. Engaging and strengthening these muscles through exercises like the Superman pose can significantly improve balance, stability, and posture. Moreover, a strong core reduces the risk of injuries that can occur through everyday activities or more strenuous exercises by supporting your spine and providing a stable center of gravity.

Performing the Superman pose starts with you lying face down on a comfortable surface, arms extended in front of you, and legs stretched out behind. The simplicity of the setup belies the effectiveness of the exercise. As you lift your arms and legs simultaneously, aiming to raise them a few inches off the ground, you engage not just the lower back but the entire lineup of muscles running along your spine and core. Hold this lifted position for a few seconds, feeling the gentle pull along your back and the engagement of your abdominal muscles. It's crucial to keep your head and neck in a neutral position, aligned with your spine, to avoid any strain. Exhale as you gently lower your limbs back to the starting position, and allow yourself a moment to relax before repeating the movement.

Integrating the Superman pose into your daily or weekly fitness routine can be highly beneficial, particularly if you balance it with other core exercises that focus on different aspects of the core muscles. For instance, incorporating exercises that focus on the obliques or lower abdominals can provide a comprehensive core strengthening regimen that supports overall body health and fitness. However, it's essential to approach this integration with mindfulness. Start with a few repetitions, perhaps two to three sets of three to five lifts, and gradually increase the number as your strength and endurance improve. Listen to your body's responses. If you feel any discomfort beyond the typical muscle fatigue associated with a good workout, consider adjusting your form or reducing the intensity to accommodate your body's needs.

Safety is paramount when performing any exercise, and the Superman pose is no exception. Because this pose significantly engages the back muscles, it's essential to ensure that you're performing it correctly to avoid any potential strain or injury. One common mistake is lifting the limbs too high, which can put unnecessary pressure on the lower back. Instead, focus on lifting just enough to engage the muscles effectively while maintaining comfort. It's also helpful to keep your movements smooth and controlled; avoid jerky or rushed motions that can lead to muscle pulls. If you have pre-existing back issues, it may be wise to consult with a physical therapist or a fitness professional who can help modify the exercise to suit your specific conditions.

By incorporating the Superman pose into your routine, you not only build physical strength but also cultivate a sense of inner power and resilience. Each time you perform the pose, you are reminded of your body's capabilities and its incredible potential for growth and strength. This exercise, while simple, is a profound practice of celebrating and nurturing the superhero within, gently guiding you toward a stronger, more balanced self.

2.5 Calf and Thigh Stretches for Mobility

Imagine a day filled with ease in movement, where walking up a flight of stairs, bending to tie your shoes, or even a leisurely stroll feels effortless. This isn't just a daydream for the athletically gifted; it's within your reach through the simple practice of calf and thigh stretching. Mobility in the legs is a cornerstone of physical health, significantly affecting how freely and comfortably you can move through life. Calf and thigh muscles are pivotal in almost every motion you undertake, from standing up to sitting down, walking to running. When these muscles are tight, they can lead to discomfort, reduced mobility, and even a higher risk of injuries. By engaging in regular stretching exercises targeted at these areas, you enhance not only your flexibility but also your body's functional capabilities.

Let's delve into some accessible stretches that focus specifically on the calves and thighs, designed to be doable for anyone regardless of their fitness level. For the calves, a simple yet effective stretch is the wall push-up. *Facing a wall, extend one leg straight behind you, heel pressed to the floor, and the other leg bent in front of you. Push gently against the wall until you feel a stretch in the calf of the extended leg.* This stretch is not only easy to perform but also highly effective in lengthening the calf muscles, which are crucial for ankle mobility and overall leg function. For the thighs, the standing quad stretch provides significant benefits. Stand on one foot, using a wall or a chair for balance if needed, and pull the opposite foot towards your buttock, keeping your knees together and your back straight. This stretch targets the quadriceps, which are key players in knee health and overall thigh flexibility.

Integrating these stretches into your daily routine brings numerous benefits. Regular leg stretching can significantly improve blood circulation, which is vital for muscle health and efficiency. Enhanced circulation means more oxygen and nutrients delivered to your muscles, which helps in muscle repair and growth. Moreover, routine stretching helps reduce muscle tightness, which can be a source of discomfort and can limit your range of motion. Over time, as your legs become more flexible, you'll likely notice a decrease in day-to-day discomfort, especially in activities that involve a lot of leg use. Additionally, flexible muscles are less prone to injuries, which means you can enjoy your daily activities with a reduced risk of muscle strains or tears.

Adapting these stretches to fit different fitness levels and mobility ranges ensures that everyone can benefit from them, making this practice an inclusive part of somatic exercises. It's important to remember that each body is unique, and flexibility varies from person to person. If you find a particular stretch too challenging, there are always modifications you can make. For example, if the standing quad stretch is difficult, you can perform it while lying down, which might be more comfortable and manageable. Similarly, if extending the leg fully during the calf stretch is too intense, try bending the knee slightly to reduce the stretch intensity. These modifications allow you to benefit from the stretches without pushing your body beyond its comfortable limits.

As you continue to explore and integrate calf and thigh stretches into your somatic practice, consider the subtle ways these movements enhance your mobility and quality of life. Each stretch is not just a step toward greater flexibility but also a stride toward a more active and enjoyable life. Whether you're looking to improve your performance in sports, reduce your risk of leg injuries, or simply make day-to-day movements more comfortable, these leg stretches offer a simple and effective solution. They are a testament to how small practices can make significant changes in your physical well-being, providing a foundation for a healthier and more active lifestyle. As you progress in these exercises, observe the changes not only in your physical capabilities but also in your overall sense of well-being—how much more you can enjoy your movements and how much more connected you feel with your body's natural rhythms and capabilities.

2.6 The Side Corpse Pose: Releasing Tension from the Body

When life's pace overwhelms, finding moments to pause and deeply relax isn't just a luxury—it's a necessity for maintaining balance and health. The Side Corpse Pose, a gentle yet profoundly relaxing posture, offers a sanctuary where you can lay down the weight of the day and reconnect with the calmness of your inner world. This pose, although simple in its execution, is a powerful tool for releasing tension and fostering a deep sense of peace throughout your body.

Understanding the Side Corpse Pose begins with recognizing its roots in restorative yoga, where the focus is on positions that encourage relaxation and recovery. Unlike more active poses, the Side Corpse Pose allows complete relaxation, making it particularly beneficial for those who carry stress and tension not just in their minds but also physically in their bodies. To practice this pose, find a quiet, comfortable space where you can lie down undisturbed. *Place a yoga mat or a soft blanket on the floor to cushion your body. Lie on your side, gently extending your legs and stacking your hips in a straight line to avoid any twisting of the lower back. Rest your head on your arm or a pillow, allowing your neck to remain neutral and relaxed. Extend your top arm along the length of your body or place it comfortably on your side, whichever feels more natural and relaxing. Close your eyes, breathe deeply,*

and allow gravity to help release the tension from your muscles and joints.

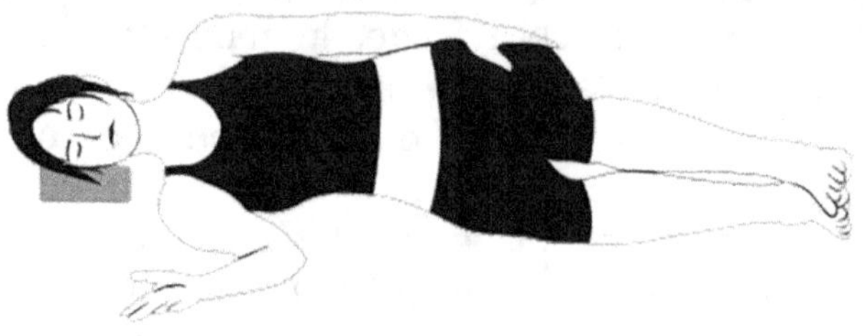

The benefits of practicing the Side Corpse Pose are both immediate and cumulative. Physically, it helps to decompress the spine and relax the muscles, particularly those along the sides of your body which can become tight from daily activities like sitting or standing for long periods. The pose encourages a deep relaxation response throughout the body, leading to reduced muscle tension and a soothing of the nervous system. Mentally, it allows for a quiet mindfulness, where you can gently observe your thoughts and sensations without attachment, helping to reduce stress and anxiety. Over time, regular practice of this pose can improve your body awareness, teaching you to notice areas of tightness or discomfort that you may typically overlook during busier moments of your day.

Incorporating the Side Corpse Pose into your relaxation and somatic exercise routines can transform your experience of downtime, turning it into a truly restorative practice. Consider creating a ritual around this pose, perhaps at the end of your day or after other forms of exercise. Use soft lighting, perhaps some calming music or natural sounds, and allow yourself at least five to ten minutes to fully engage with the pose. This practice not only enhances the physical and mental benefits but also sets a tone of intentional relaxation that can help deepen the effects of the pose on your stress levels and overall well-being.

As with any exercise, practicing the Side Corpse Pose correctly and safely is crucial to gaining the most benefit without risk of discomfort or injury. Ensure your body is aligned neutrally, with no twisting or straining, especially in the spine or neck. Use cushions or blankets to support any areas that feel strained or uncomfortable, and focus on maintaining a smooth, even breath to facilitate deeper relaxation. If you have specific health conditions or concerns, it's wise to consult with a healthcare provider or a yoga practitioner who can help you adapt the pose to suit your needs safely.

As you continue to explore the varied landscape of somatic exercises, the Side Corpse Pose stands out as a gentle yet powerful practice, ideal for those times when you need to unwind and release the burdens of stress. It's a reminder that sometimes, the most profound healing comes not from doing more, but from a deliberate and mindful stillness. Embrace this pose as a gift to yourself, a moment of peace in the midst of life's storms, and watch as its benefits permeate both your physical and emotional realms, bringing with them a renewed sense of calm and rejuvenation.

As we close this chapter on beginner-friendly somatic exercises, remember that each pose and stretch offers a unique pathway to greater health and harmony. From spine stretches that enhance flexibility and posture to the calming depths of the Side Corpse Pose, these practices are designed to meet you where you are, providing tools to support your journey toward a more balanced and vibrant life. In the next chapter, we'll explore the realm of somatic practices deeper, building upon these foundations to enhance resilience and foster an even greater connection with your body's innate wisdom.

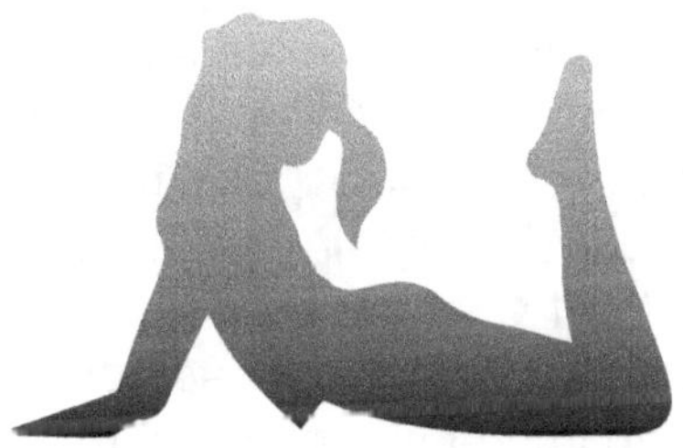

Chapter 3: *Enhancing Flexibility and Posture*

icture this: you're moving through your day with ease, each step light and unburdened, each movement fluid. It's not just a fleeting moment of grace; it's your new reality, thanks to the newfound flexibility and improved posture you've cultivated through somatic exercises. This chapter is dedicated to deepening your understanding of how targeted movements can significantly enhance your life's quality by improving your flexibility and posture. Here, we explore exercises that not only alleviate discomfort but also enrich your overall well-being, allowing you to engage with life more fully and joyously.

3.1 Pelvic Tilts for Lower Back Relief

Foundation of Pelvic Health

The pelvis: it's the keystone of your spinal health, a crucial element in the architecture of your body that affects everything from your posture to how comfortably you can sit, stand, or walk. Understanding the role of the pelvis in maintaining spinal health is essential, especially if you experience lower back discomfort. This region acts as a basin that supports your spine and core, integrating the movements of your upper and lower body. When your pelvic health is compromised, it can lead to a cascade of issues, most notably lower back pain, which affects an immense portion of the population at some point in their lives. Pelvic tilts, a gentle yet powerful somatic exercise, are designed to strengthen this foundational area, promoting alignment and easing tension in the lower back.

Executing Pelvic Tilts

Performing pelvic tilts involves a simple motion that brings profound results. *Begin by lying on your back with your knees bent and feet flat on the floor, arms by your sides.* This starting position is crucial as it provides stability and prepares your body for the movement. *Inhale deeply, and as you exhale, gently arch your lower back, pressing your pelvis upwards toward the ceiling.* You'll feel your lower back pressing into the floor. Hold this tilt for a few seconds, then slowly return to the starting position. When performed regularly, this exercise can be incredibly effective in mitigating lower back pain and strengthening the core muscles that support your spine.

Integrating into Daily Routine

Incorporating pelvic tilts into your daily routine can be done with ease and doesn't require setting aside large chunks of time. Consider integrating these exercises into your morning routine; just a few minutes each day can contribute significantly to your spinal health. Alternatively, use them as a therapeutic break from sitting at your desk or after long periods of standing. Regular engagement in pelvic tilts can help maintain your lower back's health and overall posture, making them a valuable addition to your daily activities.

Benefits Beyond Back Relief

While the immediate benefit of pelvic tilts is often felt as relief in the lower back, the advantages extend far beyond. Regularly performing this exercise can enhance your core stability, an essential element for overall strength and balance. Furthermore, pelvic tilts can improve the function of the pelvic floor, which supports several vital organs and plays a crucial role in bladder control. For women, particularly those who have experienced childbirth, strengthening the pelvic floor is integral to regaining stability and health in the pelvic region.

Interactive Element: Reflective Journaling Prompt

To deepen your connection with this practice, consider keeping a reflective journal on your experiences with pelvic tilts. After performing the exercise, take a few moments to jot down how your lower back feels compared to before the exercise. Note any changes in your posture or any reduction in discomfort. Reflecting in this way can enhance your awareness of the benefits these exercises bring to your body and encourage you to maintain this beneficial practice.

Pelvic tilts offer a simple yet effective method for enhancing pelvic health, alleviating back discomfort, and improving overall posture and body function. As you continue to integrate these movements into your daily routine, observe the subtle yet significant ways they enhance your physical health and contribute to a more vibrant, active life.

3.2 Arch & Curl: A Simple Spine Mobility Exercise

*I*magine your spine as a flexible rod that supports and moves with you through every twist, bend, and turn. Now, consider how vital maintaining that flexibility is for your overall health and well-being. Spine mobility is not just about ensuring you can reach down to tie your shoelaces or stretch up to grab something from a high shelf; it's about maintaining the health of your nervous system, the alignment of your body, and the balance of your movements. The Arch & Curl exercise, a beautifully simple yet effective movement, enhances this crucial spine mobility. It nurtures the spine's natural ability to arch and curl, providing a soothing massage to the vertebrae while also strengthening the muscles around your spine.

Let's walk through the Arch & Curl exercise, which you can easily practice on a yoga mat or any comfortable, flat surface. *Begin by lying on your back, knees bent, feet flat on the floor, arms resting by your sides, palms facing down.* This starting position is crucial as it ensures your spine is neutrally aligned with the floor, providing a safe base for the movement. *Inhale deeply, and as you exhale, gently arch your lower back, pushing your belly towards the ceiling while keeping your hips on the ground.* This creates a slight curve in your lower spine, a gentle arch that stretches and activates the muscles along your back. *After holding this arch for a few seconds, inhale and smoothly transition into the curl: pull your belly button towards the floor, flattening your lower back against the mat.* This movement should feel like a gentle hug to your spine, releasing any tension held in the muscles.

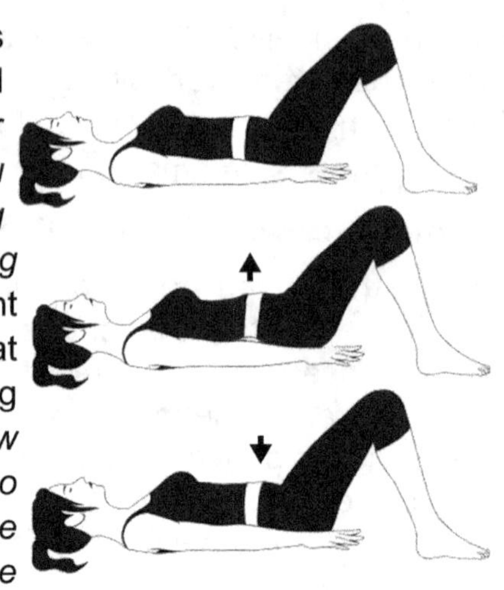

Incorporating this exercise into your daily routine can be both a meditative practice and a physical health regimen. The Arch & Curl is especially beneficial when performed in the morning as it wakes up the spine, preparing it for the day's tasks. Alternatively, using it as a tool to unwind after a long day can help alleviate the physical and mental stress that tends to accumulate. Regular practice of this exercise ensures that your spine remains agile and healthy, which can significantly improve your posture and reduce the risk of back pain, a common ailment in today's sedentary lifestyle.

Moreover, the Arch & Curl exercise beautifully complements other somatic practices by preparing the body with its foundational spinal alignment and flexibility. For instance, when paired with exercises like the pelvic tilts or the Cat Cow pose, it enhances the effectiveness of these movements by ensuring the spine moves fluidly and comfortably. This synergy not only maximizes the physical benefits but also deepens your connection to your body's movements and sensations, fostering a holistic approach to health that somatic exercises strive to achieve.

Integrating the Arch & Curl into your somatic routine encourages a dialogue between your body and mind, where each curl and arch teaches you a little more about the language of your spine. As you become more fluent in this language, you might find a deeper sense of awareness and appreciation for the incredible support your spine provides every day. This exercise, in its simplicity and effectiveness, is a testament to how small, thoughtful movements can make profound changes in your health and quality of life. As you continue to practice, let each arch and curl bring you closer to a state of balance and harmony within your body, enhancing not just your physical flexibility but also enriching your life's experiences.

3.3 Cat Cow Pose: Harmonizing Movement and Breath

The subtle art of combining breath with movement in the Cat Cow pose creates a dance between your body and mind, enhancing not just your physical flexibility but also nurturing a profound sense of inner calm. This pose, often one of the first taught in yoga classes, is not merely a physical exercise; it is a doorway to deeper body awareness and a practice in mindfulness. The Cat Cow pose offers a gentle yet powerful way to connect with the rhythms of your breath and the movements of your spine, each motion flowing into the next, creating a wave-like rhythm that massages the spine while engaging the core muscles.

To begin practicing the Cat Cow pose, position yourself on all fours on a comfortable mat. Ensure your wrists are directly under your shoulders and your knees are under your hips, setting a strong foundation for the movement. This

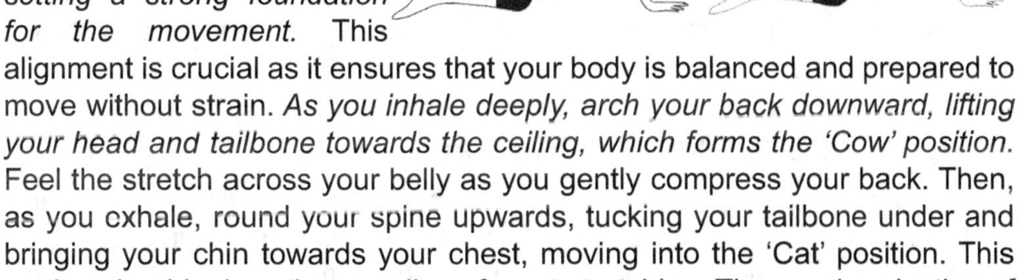

alignment is crucial as it ensures that your body is balanced and prepared to move without strain. *As you inhale deeply, arch your back downward, lifting your head and tailbone towards the ceiling, which forms the 'Cow' position.* Feel the stretch across your belly as you gently compress your back. Then, as you exhale, round your spine upwards, tucking your tailbone under and bringing your chin towards your chest, moving into the 'Cat' position. This motion should mirror the rounding of a cat stretching. The synchronization of your breath with each movement is key: inhaling as you open up into Cow, and exhaling as you round into Cat.

This fluid motion between Cat and Cow poses not only enhances the flexibility of your spine but also strengthens your core, which is essential for overall stability and balance. Each movement in the pose helps to loosen the spine, reducing stiffness and encouraging better spinal health. Moreover, the engagement of the abdominal muscles as you move between poses helps strengthen the core, which supports the spine. The rhythmic nature of the pose, guided by your breath, enhances coordination and fosters a deeper sense of body awareness. As you become more attuned to the sensations in your body with each movement, you develop a closer relationship with your physical self, learning to listen to its needs and respond with care.

Engaging in the Cat Cow pose as a mindfulness practice can transform the exercise from a simple physical activity into a meditative experience. As you flow between Cat and Cow, focus deeply on the sensations each movement brings. Notice the feeling of your muscles stretching and contracting, the way your spine moves, and how each breath fills and leaves your body. This awareness brings a mindfulness aspect to the practice, making it not just about physical movement but also about being present in the moment, connected with your body. It's a practice in living fully in the now, which can help reduce stress and increase mental clarity.

Incorporating the Cat Cow pose into your daily routine lays a foundation for greater flexibility and improved posture. Making it a regular part of your morning routine, perhaps incorporating it into your wake-up stretching, can energize your body and prepare you for the day ahead. Alternatively, using it as a way to unwind in the evening can help relieve the tension of the day and calm your mind before sleep. The versatility of the exercise makes it a valuable addition to your toolbox of wellness practices, adaptable to your needs and schedule.

As you continue to integrate the Cat Cow pose into your life, observe the subtle yet significant shifts in your physical health and your mental well-being. This pose is more than just a stretch; it's a gesture of kindness to your body, a way to harmonize your movements and breath, and a step towards a more mindful, health-focused way of living. Each time you come to your mat to practice, you're not just training your body; you're nurturing a deep, loving connection with yourself.

3.4 Wall Butterfly Pose for Hip Opening

*O*pening your hips can feel like opening a door to improved health and vitality, where each step flows more freely, and sitting feels less strained. The hips are a central hub in your body that affect not just lower body health but also influence your overall posture and alignment. The Wall Butterfly Pose is a gentle yet effective way to enhance hip flexibility, which can be particularly beneficial if you find yourself spending many hours seated, whether it's at a desk or during a long commute. Hip flexibility is not just about achieving deeper yoga poses; it's about creating ease and balance in your daily movements and ensuring that your body's structural integrity is maintained.

Let's delve into how to perform the Wall Butterfly Pose properly, ensuring safety and maximizing its benefits. Start by sitting with your back straight against a wall, which provides support and alignment
for your spine. *Bring the soles of your feet together
in front of you, drawing them as close to your
body as feels comfortable. The closer your feet
are to your body, the deeper the stretch, but it's
important to proceed gradually and listen
to your body's cues. Let your knees fall
gently to the sides, feeling the stretch in
your inner thighs and hips. The contact with the wall helps keep your spine
from rounding, which is crucial for protecting your back during this stretch.*

Breathe deeply and hold the pose, allowing the gravity to gently deepen the stretch, without forcing your knees down. Over time, as your muscles relax, you might find your knees getting closer to the ground, which indicates increased hip flexibility.

The benefits of regularly practicing hip-opening exercises like the Wall Butterfly Pose are profound. Firstly, they can significantly reduce back pain, which often results from tight hip flexors pulling on the lower spine. By loosening these muscles, you alleviate the strain on your back, which can lead to noticeable relief from discomfort and an increase in mobility. Furthermore, hip openers improve circulation in your lower body, enhancing the blood flow to your lower limbs and promoting better overall health. This increased circulation can also speed up recovery from workouts and reduce stiffness, which is especially beneficial if you lead an active lifestyle or are looking to become more active.

Integrating the Wall Butterfly Pose into your somatic practice can greatly enhance your flexibility and contribute to a more balanced and holistic approach to your body's health. Consider making this pose a regular part of your cooldown routine after workouts, or use it as a soothing practice to unwind in the evenings. The pose is also an excellent way to break up long periods of sitting during the day; just a few minutes can help reset your posture and relieve tension. Regular practice of the Wall Butterfly Pose not only improves your hip flexibility but also helps in maintaining a healthy alignment of your pelvic area, which supports your spine and contributes to a healthier posture.

As you continue to explore the benefits of hip opening, you may notice improvements not just in your physical health but also in how you carry yourself throughout the day. Your walk might feel lighter, sitting more comfortable, and your overall movement more fluid. These changes, while they may seem subtle, can significantly enhance your quality of life, making activities you love more enjoyable and reducing the risk of pain and injury. The Wall Butterfly Pose is more than just a stretch; it's a key to unlocking greater freedom and ease in your body, supporting you in every step you take.

3.5 Seated Straddle Pose: Stretching the Legs and Back

Imagine finding a pose that stretches not just your body but also expands your ability to relax and release tension. The Seated Straddle Pose does just that, reaching into the inner thighs, hamstrings, and cradling the lower back in a stretch that feels both challenging and wonderfully liberating. This pose, while seemingly straightforward, opens up more than just the physical body; it enhances flexibility and encourages a deeper connection with the subtleties of your own physical presence. Let's explore how you can master this pose, adapt it to fit your personal flexibility level, and seamlessly integrate it into your daily somatic practice for lasting benefits.

Flexibility in the legs and back is fundamental to your overall posture and health. These areas are pivotal in supporting the core structures of your body and facilitating a range of movements from walking to bending and even standing. Tightness in these areas can lead to discomfort and restrict your mobility, impacting your quality of life. The Seated Straddle Pose specifically targets these regions, encouraging a lengthening and loosening that can significantly impact your posture and ease of movement. When you sit on the floor and extend your legs out to each side, the mere act of maintaining this position initiates a stretch that you can deepen with each exhalation. It's a foundational practice for anyone looking to enhance their flexibility, particularly if you spend many hours seated at a desk or in a car, where your legs and back are prone to stiffness.

Mastering the Seated Straddle Pose requires attention to form and an understanding of your body's current boundaries. *Start by sitting with your legs as wide apart as comfortably possible and your toes pointing upwards. Keep your spine straight and tall, imagining a string pulling you up from the top of your head. This alignment is crucial as it prevents unnecessary strain on your back. Lean forward from the hips, not the waist, to keep the spine elongated rather than curved. This forward motion should be guided by your breath: inhale to prepare, and exhale as you ease deeper into the stretch. Your hands can rest gently on the floor in front of you, helping to support your upper body and control the intensity of the stretch.* Remember, the goal here is not to reach the floor with your chest but to find a stretch that feels challenging yet doable.

Adapting the Seated Straddle Pose for different flexibility levels ensures that this exercise is accessible and beneficial for everyone. If you're just beginning or find the stretch too intense, consider using props like yoga blocks or a folded blanket. Placing these under your knees can alleviate some of the strain and allow you to maintain the pose longer, gradually increasing your flexibility. Another adaptation is to sit up against a wall, allowing your back to rest against it. This can help maintain your upright posture without straining your back muscles, making the stretch more comfortable.

Integrating the Seated Straddle Pose into your daily routine can provide long-term benefits for your flexibility and general well-being. Consider incorporating this pose into your morning routine to awaken and stretch your body, preparing it for the day ahead. Alternatively, it can serve as an excellent way to wind down in the evening, releasing the tension accumulated throughout the day. Regular practice of this pose not only improves your flexibility but also enhances your mindfulness and connection to your body. As you spend more time in the pose, focus on your breath and the sensations in your muscles, embracing the stretch and the space it creates in your body. This mindful approach turns a simple stretch into a meditative practice, enriching your experience and deepening the benefits of the exercise.

By regularly engaging in the Seated Straddle Pose, you're not just working towards greater physical flexibility; you're also cultivating a habit that enhances your overall health and enriches your somatic practice. This pose is a testament to the power of simple, mindful movements to transform our relationship with our bodies, encouraging a deeper engagement with the physical self that supports a richer, more vibrant life.

3.6 Downward Dog: A Foundational Pose for Strength and Flexibility

The Downward Dog pose, a staple in many yoga practices, is much more than a stretch. It's a comprehensive exercise that strengthens and enhances flexibility throughout your body, making it a cornerstone of somatic practice. This pose engages multiple muscle groups simultaneously, from your arms down to your legs, while also opening up the spine and improving circulation. Its ability to foster both strength and flexibility in a single movement is what makes the Downward Dog so integral to somatic routines, providing a solid foundation for physical health and well-being.

Executing the Downward Dog with proper form and alignment is crucial for maximizing its benefits and ensuring safety. *Start on your hands and knees, with your wrists aligned under your shoulders and your knees under your hips. Spread your fingers wide on the mat, pressing firmly through your palms and knuckles. As you exhale, tuck your toes under, lift your knees off the mat, and raise your hips toward the ceiling. Straighten your legs as much as you can, keeping them slightly bent if necessary to maintain comfort. Your body should form an inverted "V" shape.* It's important to keep your head between your arms, in line with your spine, and avoid hanging it down, which can strain your neck. Press your heels toward the floor; they don't need to touch the ground, as flexibility will vary from person to person. The alignment of your arms and back should be straight, avoiding any sagging in your shoulders or arching in your lower back.

Variations of the Downward Dog can make this pose accessible for beginners and those with limited flexibility, while also providing challenges for more advanced practitioners. If you're just starting out or find the standard pose too intense, try the Puppy Pose variation where you keep your knees on the ground, stretching your arms forward and pushing your hips back towards your heels. This modification reduces the weight your arms and shoulders need to support and is gentler on your back. For those seeking to deepen their practice, incorporating a leg lift within the pose can enhance strength and balance. *While in the Downward Dog, lift one leg at a time high up towards the ceiling, keeping your hips square and your weight evenly distributed across both arms.*

Incorporating the Downward Dog into your daily routine offers numerous benefits. It can serve as a great morning stretch, awakening your body and increasing blood flow after a night's rest. Alternatively, using it as a transitional pose between more intense exercises can help maintain heat in your body and provide a moment of active recovery. Regular practice of the Downward Dog not only builds strength, particularly in your arms, shoulders, and back, but also improves flexibility in your hamstrings, calves, and the arches of your feet. Moreover, this pose helps to decompress the spine, which can relieve back pain and improve overall posture.

As you weave the Downward Dog into your somatic practices, observe the ways it enhances not just your physical state but also how it encourages a mental focus and resilience. The pose demands a balance of strength and flexibility, asking you to push through the challenges while also accommodating your body's current limits. It teaches patience and perseverance, qualities that extend beyond your mat and into daily life. As you master this pose and experience its benefits, you may find it becoming a fundamental part of your routine, a trusted tool for maintaining your physical and mental health.

As we conclude this exploration of the Downward Dog and other transformative poses in this chapter, remember each posture not only enhances specific physical capabilities but also contributes to a broader sense of well-being. These practices are designed not just to improve flexibility and strength but to deepen your connection with your body, helping you move through life with grace and resilience. As you carry these lessons onto the next chapter, keep nurturing this connection, allowing it to guide you towards a healthier, more balanced existence.

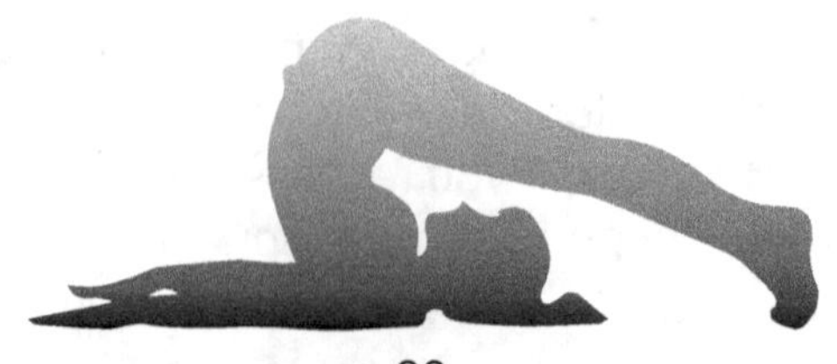

Chapter 4: *Building Strength and Toning*

Imagine feeling a surge of strength coursing through your body, not just during a workout, but in everyday moments—carrying groceries, climbing stairs, or playing with your kids. This sense of enduring strength isn't just for athletes; it's achievable for everyone, including you, through mindful and targeted somatic exercises. In this chapter, we explore how enhancing your body's strength and toning isn't merely about aesthetics but about empowering yourself to live a fuller, more active life. Let's deepen our understanding of how nurturing our body's strength fundamentally supports our overall health and wellness, especially focusing on an often overlooked but crucial aspect: the posterior chain.

4.1 The Locust Pose: Strengthening the Posterior Chain

Posterior Chain Awareness

The term "posterior chain" refers to the muscles on the backside of your body, including the lower back, glutes, hamstrings, and calves. These muscles are pivotal not only for everyday movements such as walking, standing, and bending but also for maintaining good posture and preventing injuries. Often, our lifestyle habits, particularly prolonged sitting, can lead to a weakening of these essential muscles, making us prone to discomfort and less efficient in our movements. Understanding the significance of the posterior chain and actively working to strengthen it can lead to remarkable changes in how you feel daily—imagine fewer aches, improved posture, and enhanced mobility.

Performing the Locust Pose

The Locust Pose, or Salabhasana, is a transformative exercise that specifically targets and strengthens the posterior chain. *To perform this pose, start by lying flat on your stomach on a comfortable mat, arms at your sides, and your forehead gently touching the ground. Extend your legs straight behind you, keeping them hip-width apart, and point your toes. As you inhale, gently lift your head, chest, arms, and legs off the ground. Your hands should be reaching towards your feet, palms facing each other. Imagine you are soaring through the air like a superhero* - this visualization not only adds a bit of joy to the pose but also helps in maintaining the lift. Hold this position for a few breaths, feeling the engagement in your lower back, glutes, and hamstrings. Exhale as you gently lower your body back to the mat. Repeat the pose a few times, allowing your strength to build gradually.

Benefits of a Strong Posterior Chain

The advantages of strengthening your posterior chain extend far beyond the aesthetic; they enhance your functional abilities and contribute to a healthier body alignment. A strong posterior chain can significantly reduce the risk of injuries, especially around the lower back, which bears much of the burden of everyday activities. Moreover, these muscles support the spine, and by strengthening them, you can improve your posture, which in turn can alleviate common issues such as chronic back pain and muscular imbalances. Additionally, engaging these muscles through exercises like the Locust Pose can lead to better performance in physical activities, making tasks that once seemed tiring feel much easier.

Incorporation into Regular Routines

Integrating the Locust Pose into your regular somatic routine can be highly rewarding. Consider including this pose in your morning exercise to energize your body or use it as a strengthening component in your cooldown sessions. For those new to this exercise, start with shorter holds, gradually increasing the duration as your comfort and strength improve. It's essential to listen to your body and proceed at a pace that feels challenging yet doable. Regular practice of the Locust Pose ensures that you are not only working towards a toned and strong body but also investing in a foundation that supports your overall health and vitality.

As you continue to explore and integrate strength-building exercises like the Locust Pose into your routine, you may notice a newfound sense of capability and confidence in your physical presence. This strength goes beyond the mat—it weaves into the fabric of your daily life, enhancing your movements and interactions. Remember, each time you engage in these practices, you are stepping into a stronger version of yourself, empowered and ready to embrace life's challenges with vigor and resilience.

4.2 Constructive Rest Pose for Core Engagement

Imagine a pose that not only fosters deep relaxation but also actively engages and strengthens your core, all while you are lying down comfortably. This might sound too good to be true, but the Constructive Rest Pose offers exactly that. This gentle yet effective posture is a foundational element in building core strength, which is crucial not just for physical activities but also for your daily movements and overall health. Engaging your core properly can transform the way you move and feel in your body, providing support to your spine and alleviating unnecessary strain on other muscles.

The Constructive Rest Pose is beautifully simple and remarkably effective. *To practice this pose, find a comfortable spot where you can lie down on your back. Bend your knees and place your feet flat on the floor, hip-width apart, close enough so your fingertips can just touch your heels. This position naturally aligns your spine and pelvis, reducing tension in your lower back. Let your arms rest alongside your body, palms facing up to promote an open, receptive posture. Gently engage your abdominal muscles, drawing them in towards your spine as you breathe out.* The key here is a gentle engagement; imagine you're tightening a belt around your waist just one notch. Maintain this mild contraction and breathe normally. This activation of the core muscles helps to stabilize the spine and pelvis, providing a foundation that supports your entire body.

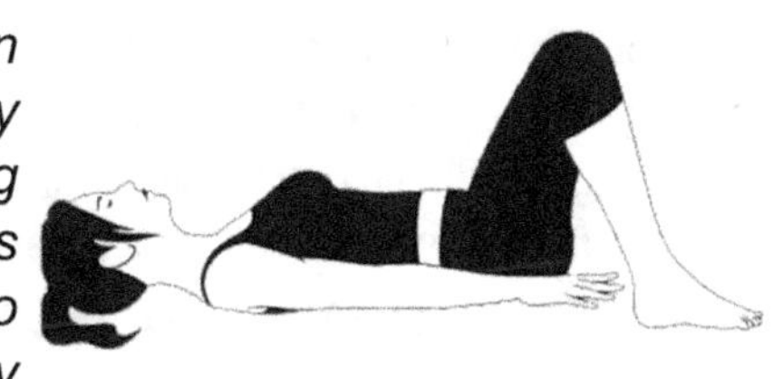

The significance of core engagement goes beyond physical appearance or strength; it's about creating a stable center from which all movements originate. A strong core reduces the risk of injuries, particularly in the lower back, which many people experience due to weak abdominal muscles. The core consists of more than just the front abdominal muscles; it includes the muscles around your trunk, sides, and back. Engaging these muscles through the Constructive Rest Pose helps to balance the muscle work around your spine, promoting better posture and reducing the strain that can lead to discomfort and pain.

Regular practice of the Constructive Rest Pose can play a crucial role in preventing lower back pain, a common ailment for many. By strengthening the core, you provide better support for your lower back, which can prevent the pain that often results from weak core muscles and poor posture. This pose is particularly beneficial because it allows you to engage your core muscles without the strain of more intense exercises that might exacerbate existing back pain. It's an accessible way to build strength right at the core of your body, ensuring that you are protecting and supporting your back with every movement you make.

Incorporating the Constructive Rest Pose into your daily routine can be seamlessly done and highly beneficial. Consider making this pose a part of your morning routine, setting a strong, stable foundation for your day. Just five minutes in the morning can help wake up your core muscles, preparing them to support you as you move through your day. Alternatively, practicing this pose in the evening can help relieve the tension that builds up from a day of sitting or standing, allowing your core and back to relax and realign. Over time, as your core becomes stronger, you might notice improvements in your posture, reduced back pain, and a greater ease in performing both everyday tasks and more strenuous physical activities.

By embracing the Constructive Rest Pose and the principles of core engagement, you are taking a significant step towards better health and a more vibrant life. This practice isn't just about building abdominal muscles;

it's about creating a harmonious balance in your body that supports your movements, enhances your posture, and enriches your overall well-being. As you continue to explore and integrate these gentle yet powerful exercises into your routine, observe the subtle yet profound ways they enhance your strength and transform your relationship with your body.

4.3 Supine Pose Crunches: A Gentle Approach to Core Strength

Imagine engaging your core in a way that not only strengthens but also nurtures your body, allowing you to feel both empowered and at ease with each movement. The Supine Pose Crunches offer this balance by focusing on gentle core strengthening that enhances your body's capabilities while being mindful of its needs and limitations. This exercise is tailored for those who might find traditional crunches too harsh or straining, providing a softer approach that still effectively engages the necessary muscles to build core strength and stability.

When performed correctly, Supine Pose Crunches focus on precision and control, avoiding the pitfalls of more aggressive exercises that can lead to strain or injury. *To begin, lie on your back with your knees bent and feet flat on the floor, hip-width apart. This starting position is crucial as it helps maintain the natural curve of your spine, preventing undue stress on your lower back. Place your hands lightly behind your head to support your neck, with your elbows wide. Inhale deeply, and as you exhale, gently lift your head, neck, and shoulder blades off the floor, focusing on pulling your ribcage towards your pelvis.* The lift should be modest, enough to feel your core muscles contracting but not so high that it strains your neck or disrupts the alignment of your spine. Hold the lift for a few seconds, then slowly lower back down, allowing your body to fully relax before the next repetition.

This nuanced approach to engaging the core helps to target the muscles effectively without the risk of injury. It's essential to keep the movement controlled and to avoid pulling on your neck, which is a common mistake. Instead, imagine a string attached to your chest pulling you upwards, which helps engage the correct muscles and preserves the integrity of your form. By adjusting the intensity of the contraction and the number of repetitions, you can customize the exercise to match your current fitness level, making it a versatile tool in your strength-building repertoire.

Integrating breathwork into your Supine Pose Crunches can significantly enhance their effectiveness and turn this physical exercise into a mindful practice. Each inhalation and exhalation can be synchronized with your movements, deepening your focus and connection with your body. As you prepare to lift, take a deep breath in, and as you curl up, exhale slowly, feeling the contraction of your abdominal muscles. This breathing pattern not only helps in performing the exercise with better form but also increases the oxygen flow to your muscles, making the exercise more dynamic and beneficial. The rhythmic breathing also aids in relaxation, ensuring that each session of crunches is as much about nurturing your body as it is about strengthening it.

Incorporating Supine Pose Crunches into a balanced somatic routine contributes to a holistic approach to fitness where strength is built without compromise to well-being. These exercises can be included as part of a daily routine, perhaps in the morning to awaken and prepare your body for the day's tasks or in the evening as a way to wind down and focus inward after a busy day. Over time, as your core becomes stronger, you'll likely notice improvements in other areas of your physical health, such as enhanced posture, reduced back discomfort, and greater ease in performing daily tasks that require core stability.

By embracing the gentle yet effective method of Supine Pose Crunches, you are making a commitment to build your strength in a way that honors your body's needs, fostering a sense of empowerment and well-being that radiates beyond the mat. As you continue to engage in these exercises, observe the subtle shifts not only in your physical strength but in your overall health and how comfortably and confidently you move through your day.

4.4 Warrior Poses: Building Strength with Balance

When you step into a Warrior Pose, you are not just lifting your arms and stretching your legs; you're embodying strength and stability, poised in balance that radiates from your core to the tips of your fingers. The Warrior Poses, known as Virabhadrasana in the yoga world, are more than physical postures; they are symbols of endurance and internal power. These poses blend the art of balance with the science of strength-building, creating a holistic approach to enhancing your physical and mental faculties. In this exploration, you'll delve into the techniques of various Warrior Poses, understanding their alignment and muscle engagement, which are crucial for safety and effectiveness. Beyond their physical benefits, these poses offer profound mental and emotional boosts, such as heightened focus and increased confidence, which can significantly impact your everyday life.

Warrior Poses require a combination of focus, breath, and alignment to execute correctly. Let's break down the technique for one of the most common - Warrior II. *Begin by standing with your feet wide apart, roughly three to four feet, depending on your height. Turn your right foot out 90 degrees, aligning the heel with the arch of your left foot, which you'll turn in about 45 degrees. As you inhale, raise your arms to shoulder height, reaching actively out to the sides, palms facing down. On an exhale, bend your right knee, aiming to get your thigh parallel to the floor, with your knee directly over your ankle. Your gaze should be directed over your right hand, embodying the focus and determination characteristic of a warrior. This alignment not only maximizes the stretch across your legs and hips but also engages your core and improves your balance.* The key is to root down through your feet, drawing energy up through your legs and torso, which helps in stabilizing your posture and strengthening your core muscles.

The physical benefits of practicing Warrior Poses are manifold. They strengthen your legs, open your hips and chest, and stabilize your core, contributing to an overall enhancement of your physical fitness. However, the benefits extend beyond the physical. These poses require and cultivate an intense focus, which can translate into improved concentration in your daily tasks. The act of maintaining balance while holding the pose also teaches physical and mental resilience, training you to remain calm and centered in challenging situations. Additionally, the powerful stance and the endurance required in these poses can boost your confidence, empowering you to feel more capable and strong, not just on your mat but in various aspects of your life.

Incorporating Warrior Poses into your regular somatic exercise routine can invigorate your practice with dynamic strength and balance training. These poses are versatile and can be modified to suit a range of fitness levels. For beginners, reducing the depth of the leg bend or practicing near a wall for support can help in slowly building the strength and flexibility required. For more advanced practitioners, adding elements like arm movements or transitions into other poses can increase the intensity of the workout, providing new challenges and opportunities for growth. Regularly practicing these poses can create a balanced routine that not only strengthens the body but also centers the mind, making your exercise regimen a truly holistic practice.

As you continue to explore and integrate Warrior Poses into your routine, observe the subtle yet profound shifts in your strength, balance, and mental clarity. Each time you step into a Warrior Pose, you are reinforcing your resilience and fortifying your focus, crafting a version of yourself that feels empowered to face life's challenges with grace and vigor. These poses are a testament to the strength that lies in balance, and the power that can be harnessed through mindful, intentional movement.

4.5 Bridge Pose for Glutes and Lower Back

When we think about the foundations of our body's strength, the glutes and lower back hold key roles that are sometimes underestimated. These areas are crucial for everyday activities like standing up from a seated position, lifting objects, or simply walking. Strengthening these areas not only boosts your overall performance but also significantly impacts your quality of life by preventing pain and injury. The Bridge Pose, a classic exercise found in both yoga and physical therapy, targets these vital areas, providing a myriad of benefits while being accessible to people of all fitness levels.

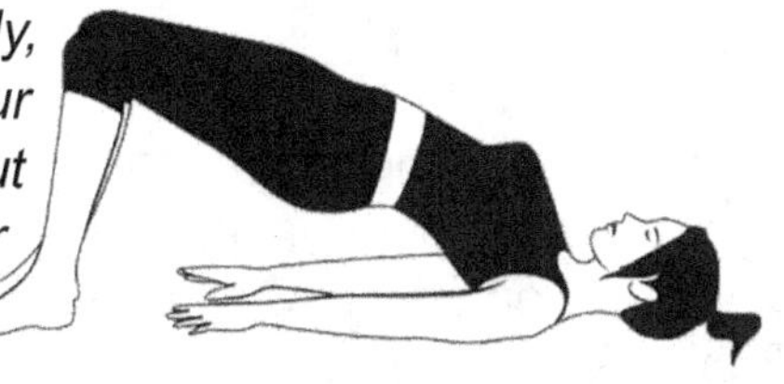

To perform the Bridge Pose effectively, begin by lying flat on your back with your knees bent and feet flat on the floor, about hip-width apart. Place your arms at your sides with palms facing down. This position sets the stage for a safe and effective lift, ensuring that the focus remains on strengthening rather than straining. As you inhale, press your feet and arms firmly into the floor and slowly lift your hips towards the ceiling. Squeeze your glutes tightly as you lift, and imagine drawing your hip bones towards your ribs, which engages your core and protects your lower back. Hold the lifted position for a few breaths, making sure your neck and shoulders stay relaxed and your spine forms a straight, diagonal line from your shoulders to your knees. To increase the challenge, you can extend one leg at a time while keeping your hips raised and stable, which intensifies the engagement in your glutes and core.

The benefits of regularly practicing the Bridge Pose extend beyond simple muscle strengthening. By activating the glutes and lower back, you are directly contributing to better posture. These muscles help stabilize your pelvis, which is crucial for alignment and balance. A well-aligned pelvis supports a healthier spine and can significantly reduce lower back pain, a common ailment that affects many. Moreover, strong glutes ensure better support for your entire body, particularly during movements that require lifting or bending, reducing the strain on other areas such as your knees and lower back.

Incorporating the Bridge Pose into your daily routine can be seamlessly done. Consider integrating this exercise into your morning routine to activate your muscles and start your day with a boost of energy. Alternatively, performing the Bridge Pose after long periods of sitting can counteract the effects of prolonged sedentary behavior by stretching and strengthening the hip flexors and lower back. Making this pose a regular part of your wellness routine not only fosters physical strength but also promotes an active and conscious engagement with your body's needs, enhancing your overall well-being.

As you continue to practice the Bridge Pose, observe the nuances of how your body responds. Each lift can bring a deeper awareness of your muscular engagements and the subtle shifts in your posture and alignment. This growing awareness is invaluable as it empowers you to take proactive steps toward maintaining your health and vitality. Engaging actively with this pose allows you to build a stronger foundation from which your body can operate optimally, turning everyday movements into opportunities for strength and renewal. As you integrate this powerful exercise into your life, appreciate the strength you are building and the positive changes it brings to your overall health and posture.

4.6 Seated Cat Cow Pose for Spinal Flexibility and Core Strength

Imagine sitting down, taking a deep breath, and simply moving in a way that brings instant relief and connection between your mind and body. The Seated Cat Cow Pose provides just that— a gentle yet profoundly effective exercise that enhances spinal flexibility and core engagement. This exercise is particularly beneficial if you find yourself sitting for long periods or if you experience stiffness in your back. It's a beautiful blend of movement and breath that nurtures your spine, strengthens your core, and rejuvenates your entire system.

To master the Seated Cat Cow Pose, start by finding a comfortable seated position on the floor or on a chair with your feet flat on the ground. If you're on the floor, cross your legs comfortably, ensuring your spine is straight and your shoulders are relaxed. Place your hands on your knees, which will help in facilitating the movement. As you inhale, arch your back slightly, pushing your chest forward and upward, and tilt your head back, opening your throat. This is the 'Cow' position, where you expose your heart and belly, inviting openness and vulnerability. As you transition into the 'Cat' position on your exhale, round your spine outward, draw your belly in, drop your head forward, and allow your shoulders to curve forward. This movement is about releasing and letting go, just as much as it is about engaging and strengthening.

This flowing movement between the Cat and Cow poses not only increases the flexibility of your spine but also strengthens your core muscles, which are vital for maintaining proper posture and balance. The rhythmic arching and rounding of your back help to lubricate the spinal discs and stretch the back muscles, alleviating tension and promoting a more fluid range of motion. Meanwhile, the engagement of your abdominal muscles as you round your back in the Cat position supports your spine and builds strength in the core, which acts as an anchor for your entire body.

Enhancing the mind-body connection is another beautiful aspect of this pose. The synchronization of your breath with the movements promotes a deeper awareness of your physical sensations and emotional state. Each inhalation and exhalation paired with the respective arching and rounding can become a mindful practice, helping you to tune into the present moment and the subtle cues of your body. This mindfulness aspect encourages a meditative state, where you can clear your mind of clutter and focus on the here and now, fostering a sense of peace and mental clarity that can carry over into your daily activities.

Integrating the Seated Cat Cow Pose into your regular somatic routine can greatly enhance your overall practice. Consider beginning your exercise session with this pose to warm up your spine and awaken your core, preparing your body for more intensive exercises. Alternatively, you can use it as a gentle cool-down sequence to relax your muscles and center your mind after a workout. It's also perfect for those moments throughout the day when you need a quick mental and physical reset. Just a few rounds can help alleviate back tension, re-energize your body, and refocus your mind, making it an invaluable tool for maintaining flexibility, strength, and mental well-being.

The simplicity and accessibility of the Seated Cat Cow Pose make it a powerful addition to your somatic practices. Whether you're a seasoned yoga practitioner or someone just starting to explore the benefits of body awareness exercises, this pose offers a gentle yet effective way to enhance your physical health and mental clarity. As you continue to incorporate this pose into your routine, pay attention to the subtle improvements in your spinal flexibility, core strength, and overall sense of well-being. Each movement, each breath, brings you closer to a state of harmony and balance, empowering you to move through life with greater ease and confidence.

As we wrap up this chapter on building strength and toning, remember that each pose and exercise shared here is a step towards a stronger, more resilient you. The Seated Cat Cow Pose, along with the other exercises explored, are more than just physical movements; they are gateways to a deeper understanding and connection with your body. By engaging with these practices regularly, you are not only enhancing your physical capabilities but also enriching your life with greater health and vitality. Let these exercises be your companions on a continuing journey towards a balanced and vibrant existence. Now, let's move forward into the next chapter, where we will explore ways to bring these practices into a cohesive daily routine, enhancing your journey towards holistic health.

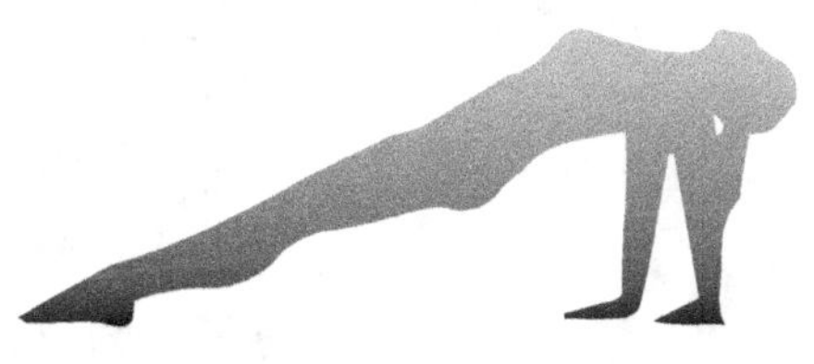

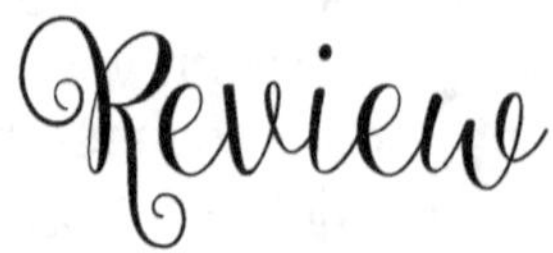

Make a Difference with Your Review
Unlock the Power of Generosity

"The best way to find yourself is to lose yourself in the service of others."

Mahatma Gandhi

My mission is to help every woman unlock their inner strength and vitality through Somatic Exercises for All Women. Everything I do stems from that mission. And, the only way for me to accomplish that mission is by reaching… well….everyone.

This is where you come in. Most people do, in fact, judge a book by its cover (and its reviews). So here's my ask on behalf of every woman who is seeking to enhance their health and happiness:

Please help those women by leaving this book a Review.

Your gift costs no money and less than 60 seconds to make real, but it can change a fellow Empowered Woman's life forever.

Your review could help...one more woman transform her life…… one more dream come true.

To get that 'feel good' feeling and help these women for real, all you have to do is... and it takes less than 60 seconds... Leave a Review.

Simply scan the QR code below to leave your review:

If you feel good about helping a fellow Empowered Woman, you are my kind of person. Welcome to the Club. You are one of us.

Your biggest fan,

L. R. Lepage,

Body Talk Practitioner and Author

Chapter 5: Practices for Emotional Awareness and Resilience

Navigating through life, we often carry more than just physical weight; our emotions also weave complex layers within us, sometimes storing tensions we are not immediately aware of. In this chapter, we delve into practices that not only illuminate these hidden emotional landscapes but also offer tools to gently release and transform them. Here, the focus is on nurturing our emotional resilience, a profound journey towards understanding and harmonizing our inner experiences with the outer world.

5.1 Body Scanning for Emotional Release

Deepening Emotional Awareness

Body scanning is a meditative practice that allows you to tune into your body, part by part, uncovering areas where emotional tension is held. Often, we are unaware of how much tension our bodies carry—tension that can be a manifestation of unresolved emotions, stress, or past traumas. By gently directing your attention to different parts of your body, you can start to recognize these tensions. This awareness is the first step towards emotional release. It's akin to turning on a light in a room that's been darkened for too long; suddenly, you can see and address what's there. This deepened awareness not only helps in identifying the sources of discomfort but also enhances your connection to your body, fostering a nurturing relationship where you learn to listen and respond to your body's needs with compassion and understanding.

Guided Steps for Emotional Release

Let's walk through a guided body scanning process designed to identify and release stored emotions. Find a quiet, comfortable place to sit or lie down. Close your eyes and take a few deep breaths, allowing your body to relax with each exhale. Start with your feet, noticing any sensations, warmth, tension, or discomfort. Gradually move your attention up through your legs, hips, abdomen, and chest—areas that often harbor emotional tension. Pay special attention to your shoulders and neck, where stress tends to accumulate. As you scan each area, imagine breathing warmth and relaxation into it, and exhale any tension or discomfort you might find. If emotions arise, acknowledge them without judgment and allow them to express themselves. This might mean feeling a rush of sadness or a spark of old anger—whatever arises, let it flow through and out with your breath. This practice can be a profound release, often accompanied by a sense of lightness and deep relaxation.

Integrating Mindfulness with Body Scanning

To enhance the emotional release during body scanning, integrate mindfulness into the practice. Mindfulness involves maintaining a moment-by-moment awareness of our thoughts, feelings, bodily sensations, and the surrounding environment. By being mindful during body scanning, you can observe your emotional responses without attachment, allowing them to surface and dissipate more easily. This integration not only deepens the emotional release but also cultivates a habit of mindfulness that can help manage stress and increase emotional resilience. As you become more practiced in mindfulness, you may find that it naturally spills over into your daily life, helping you to stay centered and calm in a variety of situations.

Regular Practice for Resilience Building

Building emotional resilience is not about never feeling negative emotions; rather, it's about developing the capacity to handle those emotions in a healthy way. Regular practice of body scanning can be a powerful tool in this process. By routinely checking in with your body and acknowledging your emotional state, you can prevent the build-up of stress and tension. It's like regular maintenance for your car; just as you wouldn't wait until your engine fails to check the oil, don't wait until you're overwhelmed to attend to your emotional health. Make body scanning a regular part of your wellness routine, perhaps starting or ending each day with this practice. Over time, you'll likely notice a greater ease in handling emotional ups and downs, a hallmark of true resilience.

Through the practice of body scanning, you engage in a dialogue with your body, learning its unique language of sensations and responses. This dialogue enriches your understanding of yourself, deepening the connection between your physical and emotional worlds. As you continue to explore and integrate these practices, you may discover profound shifts not only in your awareness but in your overall sense of well-being and balance. Each session of body scanning is an opportunity to meet yourself with kindness and curiosity, fostering a resilience that supports and enriches your life in countless ways.

5.2 Visualization for Self-Compassion and Healing

Harnessing the power of your mind through visualization is like opening a book where you are both the author and the hero of your healing journey. This practice involves picturing a scenario in your mind's eye, crafting scenes that elevate your spirit and foster profound emotional healing. Visualization isn't just about seeing; it's about feeling and believing in the transformative power of your own thoughts to shape your reality. Engaging in this practice can be a nurturing way to enhance self-compassion, allowing you to connect with yourself in a deeply affirming way, and to heal wounds from your past that may be influencing your present and future.

To begin mastering visualization techniques, consider this step-by-step approach designed to cultivate a loving and compassionate relationship with yourself. First, find a quiet, comfortable space where you won't be interrupted. Sit or lie down in a relaxed position, close your eyes, and take a few deep breaths to center yourself. Start by envisioning yourself in a place that feels safe and serene. This could be a real place you've visited before, like a beach at sunset, or somewhere imagined, like a garden filled with flowers glowing under a silver moon. Picture yourself in this space, feeling completely at peace. Now, imagine a warm, gentle light enveloping you, its glow a physical representation of love and kindness. With each breath, this light grows brighter, filling you up with a sense of unconditional self-love and acceptance. As you bask in this light, allow yourself to feel gratitude for your body, your mind, and your spirit, acknowledging your strengths and forgiving your shortcomings.

Visualization can also be a powerful tool for healing past traumas. In this practice, it's important to tread gently, acknowledging that revisiting painful memories can be challenging. If you choose to use visualization for this purpose, it might be helpful to envision yourself as you are now, offering comfort and understanding to your younger self who experienced the trauma. Picture this scene as vividly as you can: perhaps you could sit beside your younger self, offering words of comfort, understanding, and courage. You might visualize giving them a symbol of strength, like a shield, or a source of light, like a lantern, empowering them to face their fears and heal. This act of self-compassion not only helps to soothe old wounds but also reinforces your current strength and resilience.

To make visualization a daily practice, integrate it into your routine in a way that feels natural and enriching. Many find it helpful to practice visualization first thing in the morning, setting a positive tone for the day or last thing at night, allowing these healing images to marinate in the subconscious during sleep. Consistency is key—the more regularly you practice visualization, the more natural it will become, and the greater impact it will have on your emotional wellness.

Visualization is not just about escaping reality; it's about constructing a reality where healing is possible and where self-love and compassion are abundant. Each session is a step toward not only healing old wounds but also building a more resilient and compassionate self. In this safe space you've visualized, the challenges you face can be met with a new lightness and a profound sense of your own strength. As you continue to explore and engage with this practice, observe the subtle shifts in your feelings and attitudes toward yourself and the world around you. These changes, though perhaps small at first, can profoundly influence your journey toward emotional wellness and self-care, illuminating pathways to resilience that once seemed shrouded in shadow.

5.3 Mindful Walking: A Path to Emotional Balance

Imagine transforming your daily walks into sessions of profound peace and emotional balancing, where each step becomes a conscious act of moving towards greater well-being. This transformation is not only possible but can be beautifully simple through the practice of mindful walking. Often, we walk with the intention of getting from one place to another, lost in thoughts of the past or plans for the future, rarely paying attention to the act of walking itself. Mindful walking invites you to change this pattern, turning walking into a meditative practice that brings you into the present moment, helps you connect with your surroundings, and provides a gentle but powerful way to manage stress and emotions.

Mindful walking starts with intention. Before you begin your walk, take a moment to consciously decide to focus on the experience of walking. Feel your feet touching the ground, listen to the rhythm of your steps, and notice the movement of your body as you walk. With each step, mentally note the lifting, moving, and placing of each foot. You can synchronize your breathing with your steps, perhaps inhaling for three steps and exhaling for three steps, creating a rhythm that helps maintain your focus. This simple act of paying attention can turn a regular walk into a profound experience, enhancing your awareness and bringing a sense of calm and centering to your mind.

Connecting with nature during your walks can significantly enhance the benefits of this practice. Walking in a natural environment, like a park, forest, or by a body of water, can provide a sensory experience that is deeply soothing and restorative. The sights, sounds, and smells of nature can help you feel more connected to the world around you, fostering a sense of peace and reducing feelings of stress or anxiety. The natural setting can also serve as a reminder of the beauty and rhythm of the natural world, encouraging a deeper appreciation that can be calming and uplifting.

Incorporating mindful walking into your routine can be as flexible and personal as you need it to be. You might choose to take a mindful walk early in the morning, setting a serene tone for the day ahead. Alternatively, a walk during a break at work or in the evening can help you unwind and reflect. Even just a few minutes of mindful walking can be beneficial, so consider integrating this practice into your daily life in a way that feels achievable and enjoyable. Regular mindful walking can significantly improve your emotional health, helping to develop a habit that supports a balanced, mindful approach to life's challenges and stresses.

As you continue your practice, you might find mindful walking becoming a vital part of your journey toward emotional balance and well-being. Each step taken with awareness reinforces your connection to the present moment and to yourself, fostering resilience and a peaceful state of mind that can enhance all areas of your life. This practice is a gentle yet powerful way to cultivate a deeper sense of calm and clarity, one step at a time.

5.4 VOO Sound for Vagus Nerve Stimulation and Relaxation

In the realm of somatic practices, the power of sound often goes unnoticed, yet it holds a remarkable capacity to influence our physiological and emotional states. Among these, the VOO sound technique is a profound tool for engaging and stimulating the vagus nerve, which plays a critical role in our body's relaxation and healing processes. This technique, though simple in execution, can have a deep impact, promoting relaxation and fostering a sense of calm that permeates throughout the body.

The VOO sound technique involves vocalizing a deep, resonant sound that is felt as a vibration throughout your body, particularly in the chest and abdomen, areas where the vagus nerve is most accessible. To practice this technique, find a comfortable seated or lying position where you can relax without interruption. Begin by taking a deep breath into your belly, allowing it to expand fully. As you exhale, vocalize the sound 'VOO,' drawing out the sound as long as your breath allows, and focusing on feeling the vibration deeply in your body. It's important that this isn't forced; the tone should be deep, rich, and soothing. The vibration stimulates the vagus nerve, which runs from the brain through the face and thorax to the abdomen. By engaging this nerve through the VOO sound, you activate its calming effects across your body's systems, helping to reduce stress, mitigate anxiety, and enhance your overall mood.

The benefits of regular stimulation of the vagus nerve through the VOO sound are extensive. By activating this nerve, you encourage your body to move into a state of relaxation, counteracting the often overstimulated sympathetic nervous system, which is responsible for the 'fight or flight' response. Regular practice can lead to decreased anxiety levels, lower heart rate and blood pressure, and improved emotional resilience. The vagus nerve also plays a significant role in your digestive and immune systems, meaning that stimulating it can aid in digestion and bolster your immune response, contributing to overall physical health.

Incorporating the VOO sound technique into your daily practices can be both a grounding and transformative addition. This practice can be particularly effective when integrated at the beginning or end of your day, serving as a powerful bookend that helps to either prepare your body and mind for the day ahead or to unwind and process the day's events. Integrating it with other relaxation techniques, such as deep breathing or meditation, can enhance its effects, creating a deeper sense of calm and a more profound relaxation experience. As with any practice, consistency is key—the more regularly you engage in making the VOO sound, the more pronounced its benefits will become, gradually enhancing your ability to manage stress and maintain emotional balance.

As you explore the power of the VOO sound technique, allow yourself to be patient and observant, noticing the subtle ways in which it affects your body and mind. Each practice session is an opportunity to deepen your connection with your inner self, tuning into the nuances of your body's responses, and fostering a harmonious balance within your nervous system. This technique is not just about relaxation; it's about empowering yourself with tools that support your well-being in a profound and accessible way. Through regular practice, you may find a greater sense of peace and resilience, qualities that can enrich your life in countless ways.

5.5 Seated Neck Rolls: Releasing Emotional Stress

When we explore the realm of somatic exercises, it's essential to acknowledge the areas where emotional stress tends to accumulate without our conscious awareness. One such critical area is the neck and shoulders. It's not uncommon to hold tension in these parts of our bodies, which can often act as a storage space for daily stress and deeper, unresolved emotions. Seated neck rolls offer a gentle yet effective method to release this tension, fostering not only physical relief but also promoting emotional well-being.

The technique of performing seated neck rolls involves a series of simple, deliberate movements designed to gently stretch and relax the neck muscles. *To begin, find a comfortable seated position. This could be on a chair with your feet flat on the ground and your spine straight, or sitting cross-legged on the floor, whatever makes you feel stable and grounded. Start by inhaling deeply, and as you exhale, gently lower your chin to your chest, feeling the stretch along the back of your neck. Inhale as you slowly roll your head to the right, bringing your right ear close to your right shoulder, and pause to feel the stretch on the left side of your neck. Continue the motion, exhaling as you roll your head back, allowing your head to gently tilt backward and then continue inhaling as you bring the left ear towards the left shoulder. Complete the circle by exhaling and bringing your chin back to your chest. This circular motion can be repeated three to five times, and then reversed, offering balance in the muscle engagement and stretch.*

The benefits of regularly engaging in this simple exercise are profound. Each roll not only helps to loosen the muscles and increase blood flow to the neck and shoulders, thereby reducing physical tension and associated pain, but it also facilitates a release of emotional stress. The neck is a bridge between your brain - the seat of your mind - and the rest of your body. By focusing on relaxing this key area, you encourage a flow of communication and energy throughout your body, which can help to alleviate mental stress and enhance a sense of overall well-being.

Incorporating seated neck rolls into your daily routine can serve as a powerful tool for managing stress and fostering emotional balance. Consider integrating this practice into your morning routine to help loosen any stiffness from sleep and prepare both your body and mind for the day ahead. Alternatively, performing neck rolls during the day, especially if you spend long periods at a desk, can serve as a beneficial break, not only easing physical tension but also providing a mental refresh, helping to maintain productivity and focus. Additionally, concluding your day with this practice can be a soothing transition into a relaxed evening, particularly if your day has been stressful or emotionally taxing.

As you incorporate seated neck rolls into your life, pay close attention to the subtle shifts not only in your physical tension but in your emotional state as well. Over time, you may find a noticeable decrease in your overall stress levels and an increase in your emotional resilience. This practice isn't just about moving your neck; it's about understanding and nurturing the connection between your physical posture and your emotional landscape. Each rotation offers an opportunity to let go of the old stresses and invite in a renewed sense of peace and balance, making seated neck rolls a simple yet profound addition to your repertoire of self-care practices.

5.6 Shoulder Rolls: Easing Tension and Anxiety

In our daily lives, the shoulders often become a repository for stress and tension, mirroring the burdens we carry both physically and emotionally. Shoulder rolls, a simple yet profoundly effective exercise, target this area to release accumulated stress, providing both physical and emotional relief. This gentle movement can serve as a quick intervention to alleviate shoulder tension which often contributes to overall anxiety and discomfort.

The process of performing shoulder rolls is straightforward yet requires attention to detail to ensure maximum benefits. *Begin by sitting or standing in a relaxed posture. Let your arms hang loosely at your sides and focus on releasing any tension you're holding in your shoulders. Inhale deeply, and as you exhale, slowly lift your shoulders towards your ears in a gentle shrug. Continue the motion by rolling your shoulders back, feeling the shoulder blades draw together and downwards.* This backward motion opens up the chest, counteracting the forward slump that often accompanies sitting at desks or looking at screens. *Complete the circle by bringing* your shoulders forward, continuing to synchronize your movements with your breath. Repeat this cycle several times, each time focusing on the sensation of tension releasing with each roll. By engaging in this practice, you're not just loosening the muscles; you are also enhancing blood flow to the area, which can reduce muscle stiffness and promote relaxation.

Shoulder rolls stand out as a particularly effective tool for quick anxiety relief. During moments of stress or when feelings of anxiety begin to surface, performing shoulder rolls can offer an immediate calming effect. The physical movement helps to break the cycle of tension build-up, which is often a physical manifestation of stress, and encourages the release of endorphins, the body's natural painkillers and mood elevators. This makes shoulder rolls an accessible and quick method to manage stress and anxiety, especially useful when you need to regain a sense of calm swiftly.

Integrating shoulder rolls into your broader somatic practice can enhance the holistic benefits of your routines. These movements can be seamlessly incorporated into yoga sequences, warm-up routines before exercise, or relaxation sessions after a long day. By making shoulder rolls a regular part of your practice, you not only address the immediate areas of tension in the shoulders and neck but also contribute to a broader sense of bodily relaxation and emotional balance. Regular engagement in this practice can reinforce your body's resilience against stress and improve your overall posture, which is often compromised by tension and stress.

As you continue to explore the diverse techniques within this chapter aimed at cultivating emotional awareness and resilience, the simplicity and effectiveness of shoulder rolls remind us that sometimes, the most profound changes begin with the smallest movements. Each roll not only eases physical tension but also invites a lighter, more relaxed state of being, where managing stress becomes more intuitive and grounded in body awareness. This practice, though minor in effort, plays a significant role in maintaining your emotional balance and physical health, proving that in the economy of well-being, every small investment counts.

Reflective Element: Journaling Prompt

After your next session of shoulder rolls, take a moment to jot down your experiences in a journal. Reflect on any changes in your physical sensations, particularly in areas of tension around the shoulders and neck. Note any shifts in your emotional state as well. Did the exercise bring a sense of relief? Do you feel less anxious or more relaxed? Keeping track of these observations can be incredibly insightful, helping you to better understand your body's responses to stress and relaxation techniques.

As we wrap up our exploration of practices designed to enhance emotional awareness and resilience, it's clear that the journey toward emotional balance involves a combination of awareness, action, and reflection. From body scanning to mindful walking, each technique offers a unique pathway to understanding and managing your emotions. Shoulder rolls, in particular, underscore the importance of addressing physical manifestations of stress as part of your emotional health strategy. As we transition into the next chapter, we'll delve deeper into how these practices can be integrated into a comprehensive daily routine, ensuring that the benefits of what you've learned can be woven seamlessly into the fabric of your everyday life. This ongoing integration is key to building a resilient, aware, and balanced self.

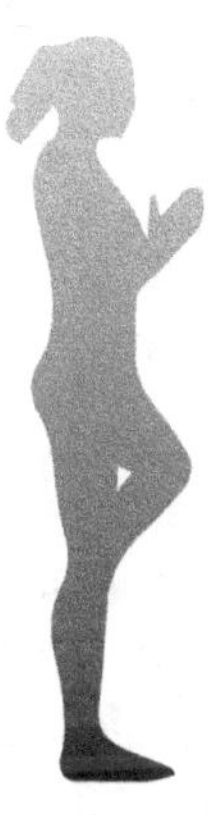

Chapter 6: Clearing Stagnant Energy and Enhancing Vitality

Imagine waking up each morning feeling lighter, as if a weight has been lifted, not just from your shoulders but from your very spirit. This sense of renewal isn't just a fleeting moment but a profound transformation that can be achieved through the art of clearing stagnant energy. In this chapter, we explore the potent practice of Emotional Freedom Techniques (EFT), commonly known as tapping. This technique isn't just about physical touch; it's a journey into the depths of your emotional landscape, unlocking and releasing the energies that hinder your vitality and cloud your emotional clarity.

6.1 Tapping (EFT) for Energy Flow and Emotional Clearing

EFT Basics for Emotional Clearing

EFT, or tapping, is a transformative practice that combines the ancient wisdom of acupressure with modern psychology. The technique involves tapping specific meridian points on your body with your fingertips while focusing on particular emotional issues. This process is designed to balance the energy system of your body, which can often be disrupted by stress, leading to emotional and physical discomfort. When you tap these points, while mentally tuning into your emotional state, you're essentially sending signals to your brain to calm the stress response. Many describe the feeling as having the volume turned down on their emotional intensity, allowing clearer thinking and a greater sense of peace.

Step-by-Step EFT Tapping Process

To begin with EFT, find a quiet space where you can be comfortable and undisturbed. Start by identifying the issue you want to focus on, which could be a specific feeling, a recent stressful event, or even a physical pain. Acknowledge this issue and accept yourself despite it; this is key to the effectiveness of EFT. You might start by tapping on the karate chop point (the outer edge of your hand) while saying a setup statement aloud, such as, "Even though I have this [anxiety], I deeply and completely accept myself." After your setup, proceed to tap lightly but firmly on the sequence of points: eyebrow, side of the eye, under the eye, under the nose, chin, beginning of the collarbone, under the arm, and top of the head. While you tap each point, repeat a reminder phrase related to your issue, such as "this anxiety."

EFT for Daily Emotional Management

Incorporating EFT into your daily routine can be a game-changer in how you manage your emotions and respond to stress. It can be particularly effective when used to start your day, setting a tone of calm and clarity, or in the evening, to process and release the day's stresses. This practice is highly flexible and can be adapted to fit any schedule or need. Regular tapping can help in gradually reducing the intensity of emotions associated with past events, easing current stress, and even in preemptively managing anticipated challenges.

Integrating EFT with Other Somatic Practices

EFT can be seamlessly combined with other somatic exercises to enhance your overall emotional and energetic health. For instance, after a tapping session, engaging in a yoga sequence or a mindful walk can further enhance the flow of energy through your body, solidifying the effects of EFT. Alternatively, initiating a body scan after tapping can help you deeply tune into the nuances of your emotional and physical state, promoting profound healing and awareness. This integrated approach not only amplifies the benefits of each individual practice but also creates a comprehensive routine that supports a wide range of your wellness needs.

Reflective Element: Journaling Prompt

To deepen your understanding and tracking of EFT's impact, maintain a journal of your tapping sessions. Note the emotions or physical sensations that arise before and after tapping, any changes in your emotional intensity, and your overall sense of well-being. This reflective practice can provide insights into patterns and progress, enhancing your ability to manage your emotional landscape effectively.

By embracing EFT, you are taking a powerful step towards not only managing your emotional health but actively enhancing your vitality and clearing the pathways to your true potential. This technique, though simple, holds the capacity to transform profound layers of your emotional being, inviting a lighter, more vibrant energy into your life. As you continue to explore and integrate tapping into your daily routine, observe the shifts in your internal energy and the newfound clarity and peace that unfold.

6.2 Grounding Practices for Emotional and Energetic Stability

Grounding, often visualized as reconnecting your body to the earth, is a powerful practice that holds immense benefits for both your emotional and energetic health. In a world where it's easy to feel unmoored by daily stresses and anxieties, grounding techniques act as anchors, pulling you back from the tumult of mental overstimulation and restoring a sense of calm and stability. This practice isn't just about physical touch with the earth; it's a metaphorical grounding too, helping you to reclaim your sense of presence and connectedness. As you learn to incorporate these practices into your life, you'll find they offer a robust defense against the disorientation that often accompanies emotional overwhelm.

To understand grounding, imagine the difference between feeling scattered, with thoughts like leaves blown about by the wind, and feeling stable, like a tree deeply rooted in the soil. Grounding practices work by redirecting your energy from a flurry of thoughts and worries to a calm, centered state. You can start with something as simple as standing barefoot on grass, soil, or sand. Feel the cool or warmth of the earth beneath your feet, notice the texture, and take deep breaths to connect with your environment. This direct contact with the earth can significantly enhance your physical and emotional grounding, as the earth has a natural charge that helps neutralize stress and improve mood.

Another effective technique involves visualization, where you imagine roots growing from the soles of your feet or the base of your spine, extending deep into the earth. With each inhale, visualize drawing up stability and calm from the earth, and with each exhale, picture releasing your stress and tension into the ground. This not only helps in reducing emotional overwhelm but also reinstates a feeling of balance and connectedness with the world around you. Engaging in such visualizations can be particularly helpful when access to a natural setting is not feasible, providing a mental grounding experience that can be equally potent.

Grounding can also be a responsive technique to moments of acute emotional overwhelm. Imagine you're in a situation that triggers significant anxiety or stress—perhaps a challenging meeting or a personal interaction that stirs deep emotions. Here, grounding can be your immediate go-to tool. Techniques like focusing on the sensation of your feet in your shoes, or gently pressing your hands against something solid, or even engaging in mindful breathing can help reel your thoughts back from panic or anxiety to calmness and control. By anchoring yourself in the present moment and focusing on physical sensations, you create a buffer against the flood of overwhelming emotions, regaining your footing and your clarity.

For ongoing well-being, integrating grounding practices into your daily routine can transform your approach to handling stress and maintaining emotional stability. Start or end your day by spending a few minutes outdoors, engaging directly with natural elements, or if indoors, practicing grounding visualizations or mindful breathing. Regular grounding not only fortifies your day-to-day emotional resilience but also enhances your overall energy levels, keeping you feeling centered and ready to face whatever comes your way.

As you continue to explore these grounding practices, each step, each breath, and each moment you choose to connect with the earth or anchor yourself in the present, builds a stronger foundation for your emotional and energetic health. These practices are more than just techniques; they are invitations to experience life with a renewed sense of stability and vitality, rooted firmly in the knowledge that no matter the chaos that surrounds you, you have the tools to remain centered and grounded.

6.3 PMR (Progressive Muscle Relaxation) for Deep Relaxation

Progressive Muscle Relaxation (PMR) is a technique that teaches you to relax your muscles through a two-step process: systematically tensing particular muscle groups and then releasing the tension to notice how the muscles feel when relaxed. This practice is deeply rooted in the understanding that physical relaxation can lead to a state of mental calmness. It's particularly beneficial for those who carry emotional tension daily, manifesting as physical tightness. PMR not only aids in releasing this built-up tension but also contributes significantly to improving the quality of sleep and overall emotional equilibrium.

To begin practicing PMR, it's best to find a quiet, comfortable place where you won't be disturbed. Lie on your back with your legs uncrossed and arms relaxed at your sides, unless otherwise specified. Start by taking a few deep breaths, inhaling through your nose, and exhaling through your mouth to initiate a state of relaxation. Then, focus on each muscle group, starting either from your feet and moving upwards, or from your head down, depending on your preference. For each muscle group, engage in a cycle of tensing the muscles as you breathe in for about five seconds, and then relax them completely as you breathe out. As you release the muscle tension, imagine the stress and tension leaving your body, and focus on the sensation of relaxation. This process can be particularly enlightening, as you may discover areas of tension you were not previously aware of, offering insights into where you hold your stress.

The benefits of PMR extend beyond mere relaxation. For individuals dealing with emotional stress or those who find it difficult to unwind before sleep, PMR can be a game-changer. The methodical tensing and relaxing of muscles can decrease overall arousal and lead to deeper sleep. For those who experience insomnia due to anxiety or stress, incorporating PMR into your nightly routine can help transition your body into a state of restfulness, making it easier to fall and stay asleep. The technique's focus on physical relaxation also aids in emotional release, as reducing physical tension can help alleviate psychological stress, fostering a peaceful mind and a relaxed body.

Incorporating PMR into your evening routine can transform your approach to rest and recovery. Consider setting aside time before bed to practice PMR, perhaps after a warm bath or a light bedtime reading session. This practice can serve as a signal to your body and mind that it's time to slow down and prepare for sleep. Over time, this routine can help recalibrate your body's sleep cycle and emotional resilience, making relaxation and sleep more accessible and restorative.

As you integrate PMR into your life, observe the subtle changes not only in your sleep patterns but also in your daily stress levels and reactions to emotional triggers. This practice, while simple, offers profound benefits that enhance your ability to engage with life from a place of greater calm and less reactivity. Each session of PMR is an opportunity to deepen your connection to your body, understand your stressors, and cultivate a powerful form of self-care that supports both your physical and emotional health. As you continue on this path, let the gentle rhythmic pattern of tensing and relaxing become a trusted method for nurturing your well-being, enhancing your vitality, and restoring your spirit.

6.4 Nutrition Tips to Support Somatic Practices

Navigating the intricate relationship between our bodies and the foods we consume reveals much about our overall well-being and emotional health. In the sphere of somatic practices, where the focus is as much on emotional balance as on physical health, integrating thoughtful nutrition strategies can significantly enhance the benefits of each movement and meditation. The foods we eat play a pivotal role in supporting not just our physical body but also our emotional landscape, providing the necessary nutrients that affect our mood, energy levels, and even our perception of stress and pain.

Understanding the role of nutrition in emotional health begins with acknowledging how certain foods can influence our brain chemistry and stress responses. For instance, complex carbohydrates found in whole grains help facilitate the production of serotonin, a neurotransmitter that promotes a feeling of well-being and relaxation. On the other hand, lean proteins such as turkey, fish, and chicken contain amino acids like tryptophan, which not only help stabilize mood but also aid in the synthesis of serotonin. Incorporating a balanced diet rich in these nutrients can help enhance the calming effects of your somatic practices, making it easier to achieve a state of relaxation and maintain it. Moreover, omega-3 fatty acids, prevalent in fish like salmon and in flaxseeds, are known for their anti-inflammatory properties and their role in brain health, which can support cognitive function and emotional regulation.

Discovering specific foods and nutrients that support emotional well-being involves tuning into your body's responses to different foods and observing how they affect your energy and mood. Foods high in magnesium, such as leafy greens, nuts, and seeds, are known for their ability to help manage cortisol levels, a hormone closely linked to stress. Including these foods in your diet can provide a natural way to help manage stress, complementing your somatic exercises like yoga or mindful walking, which also aim to reduce stress levels. Additionally, antioxidants found in berries, artichokes, and dark chocolate can protect your body at a cellular level against oxidative stress, which not only impacts your physical health but can also affect your emotional state. By consciously incorporating these foods into your meals, you are not just nourishing your body but also supporting your emotional and energetic stability.

Integrating these nutritional strategies with your somatic work offers a holistic approach to emotional health, where diet and movement support and enhance each other. Consider starting your day with a breakfast rich in complex carbohydrates and proteins to stabilize your mood and energy levels, making morning somatic practices more focused and effective. Similarly, including a small portion of dark chocolate or a handful of nuts in your afternoon snack can provide the antioxidants and magnesium needed to help manage afternoon stress, enhancing the relaxation effects of any midday or evening somatic routines.

Mindful eating practices can further deepen the connection between nutrition and somatic exercises, enhancing the emotional benefits of both. Mindful eating involves paying close attention to the experience of eating— observing the colors, smells, textures, and flavors of your food, and noticing the physical and emotional sensations during and after eating. This practice not only helps in building a deeper appreciation for your food but also promotes better digestion and satisfaction with meals. By eating mindfully, you become more attuned to your body's hunger and satiety signals, which can prevent overeating and the discomfort that might distract from or hinder your somatic practices. Moreover, mindful eating can be a form of meditation in itself, providing an opportunity to practice stillness and presence, which are core aspects of somatic exercises.

As you continue to explore and integrate these nutrition tips into your daily routine, you may find that they not only enhance your somatic practices but also contribute to a more balanced and harmonious lifestyle. Each meal becomes an opportunity to support your body's needs, complementing the work you do on the mat or in your meditation space. This holistic approach not only deepens your somatic practice but also enriches your overall experience of health and well-being, allowing you to engage with life's challenges with greater ease and resilience.

6.5 Constructive Rest Pose with Cactus Arms for Open Energy Channels

Opening your energy channels can sometimes feel like a delicate dance between maintaining comfort and encouraging flow throughout your body. The Constructive Rest Pose, particularly when combined with cactus arms, serves as a gentle yet powerful tool to facilitate this balance, nurturing an open pathway for energy and enhancing your vitality. This pose, rooted in the principles of restorative yoga, is a welcoming haven for anyone, especially if you find more dynamic forms of exercise challenging due to physical constraints or personal comfort. It's about finding a sweet spot where relaxation meets energetic rejuvenation, allowing you to tap into your body's natural healing capabilities.

To embrace the full benefits of the Constructive Rest Pose with cactus arms, *start by lying flat on your back on a comfortable surface, preferably a yoga mat or a padded carpet. Bend your knees and plant your feet flat on the ground, hip-width apart, ensuring that your spine maintains its natural curve - a gentle acknowledgment of its innate structure. Let your arms fall open to the sides, bending your elbows to form a roughly 90-degree angle, resembling the shape of a cactus.* This positioning of the arms not only opens up the chest and shoulders - areas often burdened by tension and stress - but also enhances the flow of energy across these vital points. *As you settle into the pose, close your eyes and take a few deep, soothing breaths. With each exhale, envision releasing any stagnant energy that might be lurking within your body, clearing the way for fresh, vibrant energy to flow through.*

The benefits of this simple yet profound pose are manifold. By opening the chest and shoulders, areas where emotional stress is often held, the pose encourages emotional as well as physical release, fostering a sense of openness and peace. This release is not just about letting go of the bad; it's about making room for new, positive energy to enter and rejuvenate your spirit. Additionally, the grounding nature of the pose, with your back in contact with the earth, promotes a sense of stability and connectedness, providing a foundation upon which you can rebuild and refresh your energy stores. The alignment and gentle pressure on the spine also stimulate the nervous system in a subtle, calming manner, further enhancing your body's resilience and vitality.

Incorporating the Constructive Rest Pose with cactus arms into your daily routine can be a game-changer, especially when it comes to managing energy levels and maintaining emotional health. Consider making this pose a part of your morning routine to set a calm, grounded tone for the day. Alternatively, it can serve as an excellent transition into the evening, helping to dissolve the day's stresses and prepare your body and mind for a restful night. This practice doesn't demand much time - just a few minutes can have a profound impact. It's about quality, not quantity; even short sessions can significantly enhance your sense of well-being and vitality.

Combining this pose with specific breathing techniques can amplify its effects, turning a simple pose into a powerful tool for energy and emotional management. Try incorporating a deep, diaphragmatic breathing pattern while in the pose. Inhale deeply, filling your belly and chest with air, and exhale slowly, imagining a wave of relaxation sweeping through your body. This type of breathing enhances the oxygen flow to your tissues, boosting energy levels and further facilitating the release of tension and stress. As you breathe deeply in the Constructive Rest Pose, you're not just resting; you're actively participating in your own process of healing and rejuvenation.

As you continue to explore and integrate this pose into your life, observe the subtle yet significant shifts in how you feel—energetically, emotionally, and physically. Each session is an opportunity to deepen your connection with your body, to listen to its needs, and to respond with care and intention. This practice is not just about achieving a temporary sense of relaxation; it's about cultivating a sustainable, vibrant flow of energy that supports your overall health and enriches your life. Let each breath and each moment in the pose be a gentle reminder of your body's capacity for self-restoration and vitality.

6.6 Butterfly Pose A: Stimulating Energy Flow in the Pelvis

The pelvic region, often overlooked, is a pivotal area for both physical and emotional health. Its well-being is crucial because it serves as a base for your spine and a nexus for nerves that affect the lower half of your body. The Butterfly Pose A, or Baddha Konasana, targets this essential area, encouraging an open, fluid energy flow that can transform how you feel physically and emotionally. This pose helps to relieve tightness in the hips and groin, which are common areas where stress and emotions are stored. By engaging in this pose, you're not only enhancing your flexibility but also facilitating a release of emotional and energetic blockages that might be holding you back.

To perform Butterfly Pose A correctly, begin by sitting on a comfortable, flat surface. Bring your feet together, with your knees bent out to the sides, forming a diamond shape with your legs. Hold your feet with your hands, and allow your knees to gently drop towards the ground. It's important to maintain a straight back, keeping your spine aligned and your chest open. This posture should feel comfortable; if you experience any strain, consider placing cushions under each knee for support. As you settle into the pose, focus on your breathing, inhaling deeply and exhaling slowly, allowing your body to relax further with each breath. With each exhale, imagine releasing any tension held in your pelvic area, encouraging a sense of openness and flow.

The benefits of improving energy flow in the pelvic area are profound. Physically, it enhances your flexibility and eases tension in the lower back and hips. Emotionally, the release of tightness in this area can lead to a noticeable shift in how you handle stress and anxiety. The pelvic region is also linked with sexual health; thus, improving its energy flow can also enhance your sexual well-being, making this practice beneficial for your overall intimacy and personal relationships. Furthermore, the emotional release facilitated by Butterfly Pose A can lead to greater emotional stability, as it encourages the release of deep-seated emotions that may be impacting your mood and emotional responses.

Integrating Butterfly Pose A into your somatic routines can create a comprehensive approach to your emotional and energetic health. Consider beginning your practice with this pose to open up the body and establish a foundation of flexibility and emotional openness. Alternatively, use it as a closing pose to consolidate and integrate the energy work from your session. Regular practice of Butterfly Pose A can be particularly effective in maintaining and enhancing the flow of energy in the pelvic region, making it an integral part of your journey towards a balanced and harmonious body and mind.

As you continue to explore the depths of your emotional and energetic landscapes through practices like Butterfly Pose A, you forge a path to a more attuned and vibrant self. Each session is a step towards unlocking the full potential of your body's energy flow, enhancing not just your physical flexibility but also your capacity to navigate life's emotional complexities with grace and resilience. This pose, in its simplicity and effectiveness, offers a gateway to a more balanced and fulfilling experience of your body and emotions, paving the way for a healthier and more integrated self.

In summary, Chapter 6 delves into practices that not only enhance physical relaxation but also contribute significantly to emotional and energetic health. Techniques like EFT tapping, grounding practices, Progressive Muscle Relaxation, and targeted nutritional strategies work synergistically to release emotional tension, improve sleep, and support your body's natural healing processes. The introduction of Butterfly Pose A further enriches this toolkit, offering a focused method for stimulating energy flow in the pelvic region, which is essential for emotional balance and overall well-being. As we transition into the next chapter, we will explore how to integrate these practices into a cohesive daily routine, ensuring that the benefits of what you've learned are woven seamlessly into the fabric of your everyday life. This ongoing integration is key to maintaining a balanced, healthy, and vibrant lifestyle.

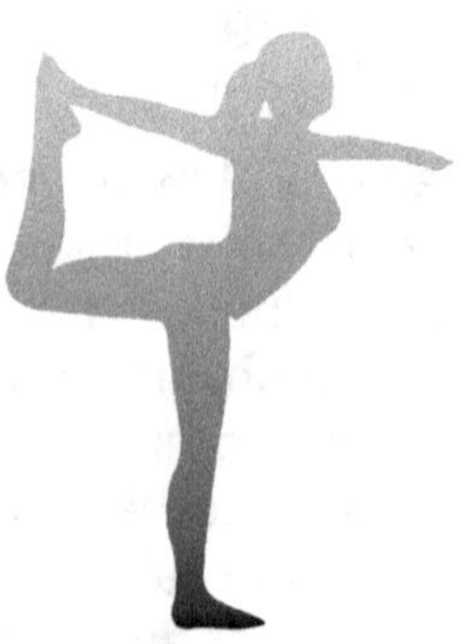

Chapter 7: Practical Tips for Daily Integration

Imagine transforming those fleeting moments throughout your workday into pockets of peace and rejuvenation. It's not just a daydream but a tangible reality that can be achieved with simple, mindful breathing techniques. In our fast-paced world, the office can sometimes feel like the least likely place for tranquility. Yet, it's exactly where such practices can have the most profound impact. By integrating mindful breathing into your daily work routine, you not only enhance your focus and productivity but also cultivate a sense of calm that can redefine your professional and personal life.

7.1 Incorporating Mindful Breathing into Your Workday

Breathing Techniques for the Office

Breathing exercises are a stealthy powerhouse—quiet and unobtrusive, yet incredibly effective at resetting your emotional state and sharpening your focus. One simple technique you can use right at your desk is the "4-7-8" breathing method. To practice this, exhale completely through your mouth, then close your lips and inhale quietly through your nose to a mental count of four. Hold your breath for a count of seven, then exhale completely through your mouth to a count of eight. This one-breath cycle can act as a mini-break, clearing your mind and reducing stress. The beauty of this exercise is its discretion—your colleagues won't even notice you're doing it, yet you'll feel the calming effects almost immediately.

Integrating Breath Breaks

Incorporating these brief breathing breaks into your daily schedule can seem daunting at first, especially when your calendar is back-to-back with meetings and deadlines. However, the key is to anchor them to certain parts of your day. Perhaps every time you finish a task, before you start another, take a two-minute breath break. Or set a reminder to practice breathing exercises every hour or so. These small pauses are like hitting a reset button for your nervous system, keeping you not just mentally but also physically refreshed.

Breathwork for Work-Related Stress

Specifically tailoring your breathwork to address work-related stress can significantly enhance your coping mechanisms. When faced with a stressful situation—be it an impending deadline or a challenging client call—utilize tactical breathing to regain control of your emotions. Tactical breathing, used by first responders and the military to stay calm in crises, involves breathing in for four counts, holding for four counts, exhaling for four counts, and holding again for four counts. This method can help stabilize your mood and bring a clear, calm perspective to any situation.

The Role of Breath in Maintaining Professional Balance

Mindful breathing does more than just alleviate immediate stress; it plays a crucial role in maintaining a sustainable balance between your professional responsibilities and personal well-being. By regularly practicing mindful breathing, you develop a resilience that buffers you against the daily pressures of work. This practice helps to cultivate a presence of mind that enhances your interactions with colleagues and improves your decision-making skills, making you a more balanced and effective professional.

As you continue to weave these breathing practices into the fabric of your daily routine, they become less of an activity and more of a natural part of your life. Each breath taken with intention is a step toward a more centered, peaceful, and resilient self. Through these practices, you are not just surviving your workday; you're thriving in it, armed with tools that transform stress into serenity and challenges into opportunities for growth.

7.2 Quick Somatic Exercises for Busy Schedules

In a world where every minute counts, finding time for extensive workout routines might often feel like a luxury you can't afford. Yet, the beauty of somatic exercises lies in their flexibility and adaptability, allowing you to weave them into the busiest of days without needing to carve out large chunks of time. Imagine being able to refresh your mind and rejuvenate your body in just five minutes or less. These quick somatic breaks can be the key to maintaining both your physical agility and mental clarity amidst a hectic schedule.

Somatic exercises tailored for those with little time to spare are designed to be both efficient and effective. For instance, a simple sequence of chair yoga can be incredibly revitalizing and requires nothing more than a chair and a few minutes. Begin by sitting at the edge of your chair with your feet flat on the floor. Engage in a series of neck rolls, shoulder shrugs, and arm stretches that release tension from the upper body, commonly accumulated from hours of desk work. Follow this with spinal twists from left to right, which not only enhance spinal flexibility but also stimulate digestion—a common concern for those who sit for long periods. Each movement flows into the next, with deep, mindful breathing linking each step. This brief session not only breaks the monotony of prolonged sitting but also boosts your circulation and refocuses your mind, making you more productive when you return to your tasks.

Furthermore, integrating these micro-practices throughout your day can transform the very rhythm of your daily life. Consider the moments you often feel your energy waning—perhaps mid-morning or during the infamous afternoon slump. These are perfect opportunities to engage in micro-somatic practices such as the 'Desk Dancer.' This involves sitting or standing near your desk and allowing your body to move freely to your favorite tune for one or two minutes. You might sway your hips, rotate your arms, or simply bob your head to the rhythm. This not only shakes off lethargy but also elevates your mood and can be a delightful way to infuse a bit of fun into your workday.

Building these practices into a habitual part of your daily routine ensures that they become second nature, just like grabbing a morning coffee or checking your emails. Start by setting specific times for your somatic breaks, perhaps aligning them with natural transitions in your day, such as after completing a major task or just before lunch. The key is consistency. Over time, these short sessions will seamlessly integrate into your daily flow, becoming a natural and integral part of your lifestyle. They serve not just as breaks but as vital components of your day that enhance your overall well-being and productivity.

Adopting quick somatic exercises into your daily routine doesn't require drastic changes—rather, it's about making small, manageable adjustments that accumulate significant benefits over time. These moments of movement and mindfulness can dramatically enhance your day, providing a quick yet effective method of stress relief, physical activity, and mental clarity. As you continue to explore and expand these practices, you may find that they not only improve your physical health but also bring a greater sense of joy and balance to your everyday life, proving that even the busiest schedules can indeed accommodate the profound benefits of somatic practice.

7.3 Using Visualization Techniques for Goal Setting

Visualization is a powerful tool that can transform your aspirations into tangible realities. It involves seeing yourself achieving your goals in your mind's eye, a practice that not only clarifies your desires but also embeds them deeply into your subconscious, enhancing your motivation and the likelihood of your success. Whether these goals are personal, like improving your health, or professional, such as advancing in your career, visualization can serve as a bridge between where you are now and where you wish to be.

The process begins with clarity. You must first clearly define what your goals are. Picture yourself having already achieved them: What does that look like? How do you feel? For instance, if your goal is to become more active and improve your health, see yourself in your ideal state of health. Visualize yourself performing somatic exercises with ease, feeling the strength and vitality in your muscles, and experiencing the joy of movement. Feel the satisfaction and the surge of health coursing through your body. The key is in the details: the more vividly you can paint this picture in your mind, the more real and attainable it will feel. This clarity not only boosts your motivation but also aligns your daily actions with your ultimate goals.

Incorporating a daily visualization practice into your routine can significantly enhance your focus and direction. Dedicate a few quiet moments each morning or evening to close your eyes and visualize your goals. This practice can be seamlessly integrated with somatic exercises; for example, while in a relaxed pose, such as the Constructive Rest Pose, you can use this time to visualize. The physical relaxation combined with mental visualization deepens the impact, embedding your aspirations into both your body and mind. Over time, this daily practice not only keeps your goals top of mind but also continually reinvigorates your drive to achieve them, turning what might sometimes feel like a distant dream into a clear, achievable vision.

Visualization also offers a powerful means to navigate and overcome roadblocks that might arise on your path to achieving your goals. When faced with a challenge, use visualization to imagine handling the situation with poise and determination. For instance, if you encounter resistance in your path, such as a lack of motivation to continue with your somatic practices, visualize yourself pushing through these barriers. See yourself completing your exercise routine and feeling exhilarated afterward. By mentally rehearsing overcoming these obstacles, you prepare yourself to face and manage them in real life with greater ease and confidence.

Understanding the synergy between somatic practices and visualization can profoundly enhance your goal achievement. Somatic exercises, which heighten body awareness and control, can be enriched with visualization to deepen emotional and physiological responses. For example, while performing a yoga pose, visualize your body becoming stronger and more flexible, aligning with your health goals. This blend of physical practice and mental imagery creates a powerful feedback loop where each element reinforces the other, accelerating your progress toward your goals.

As you continue to explore and refine your visualization techniques, remember that the power lies in consistency and belief. By regularly engaging in this practice, you deepen the mental grooves that lead to real-world success. Each session is a step toward not only seeing your goals with greater clarity but also living them with greater purpose and satisfaction. Through visualization, combined with the grounding and strengthening practices of somatics, you equip yourself with a robust toolkit for personal and professional growth, ensuring that every vision has the potential to be transformed into reality.

7.4 Nutritional Habits to Enhance Somatic Benefits

Embarking on a path where your body and mind are in tune, where every stretch and breath brings you closer to a state of well-being, is not just about the exercises you do. It's equally about the fuel you provide your body. The right nutrition can dramatically enhance the benefits of your somatic practices, transforming not just your physical health but also enriching your connection to your own body. Imagine foods acting like supportive friends, each bite not just a moment of nourishment but a step towards better body awareness and deeper engagement with your somatic routines.

Eating for somatic support involves more than just choosing healthy foods. It's about selecting nutrients that enhance flexibility, strengthen muscles, and calm the mind, directly complementing your somatic activities. Foods rich in omega-3 fatty acids, such as salmon, flaxseeds, and walnuts, are known for their anti-inflammatory properties, which can help reduce muscle stiffness and joint pain, often a byproduct of starting new physical routines. Including magnesium-rich foods like spinach, pumpkin seeds, and bananas in your diet can aid muscle relaxation and prevent cramping, making your somatic sessions more effective and enjoyable. Additionally, complex carbohydrates found in whole grains and legumes can provide sustained energy, keeping you invigorated through each stretch and pose.

Delving deeper into how specific foods can boost body awareness and connection, consider the role of antioxidants found in berries and dark chocolate. These nutrients fight oxidative stress, which can affect muscle recovery and mood. By incorporating these foods into your diet, you not only support your physical health but also enhance your sensory awareness, making you more attuned to the subtle changes in your body during your somatic practices. Hydration also plays a crucial role. Drinking enough water, infused with natural flavors like cucumber or lemon, can help maintain the fluid balance in your muscles and joints, ensuring that your movements are smooth and your body is responsive.

Integrating nutrition into your somatic routine doesn't have to be complex. Start with small, manageable changes like incorporating a smoothie rich in berries, protein, and a handful of spinach into your post-exercise routine. This not only helps in muscle recovery but also ensures you're replenishing your body with essential nutrients. Planning your meals around your somatic schedule can also enhance the benefits. For instance, a light, protein-rich meal about an hour before your practice can provide the energy you need without feeling too heavy, while a post-exercise meal with a good balance of protein and carbs can aid in recovery and prepare you for the rest of your day.

Nutrition for energy and focus is crucial, especially on days filled with activities and responsibilities beyond your somatic practices. Foods that slowly release energy, like oatmeal or quinoa, can keep you fueled for longer periods. Pair these with a good source of protein like Greek yogurt or a handful of nuts to keep your energy levels stable. Such dietary choices help in maintaining high levels of focus and stamina, which are essential not just for physical activities but for mental tasks as well. On days you practice yoga or any mindful somatic routines, consider green tea as a beverage choice. Its combination of caffeine and L-theanine can provide a smoother boost of energy and enhanced focus without the jitters associated with coffee.

As you continue to explore and refine these nutritional practices, you'll likely discover a remarkable enhancement in your overall somatic experience. Each mindful meal or snack is not just feeding your body but is actively supporting your journey towards a more connected and aware state of being. Through thoughtful nutrition, you not only empower your body to perform at its best but also deepen the very connection that makes somatic practices so transformative.

7.5 Creating a Personalized Somatic Exercise Routine

Tailoring Somatic Practices to Your Needs

When you step into the world of somatic exercises, it's like entering a garden where each path can be shaped to lead you to your own special corner of peace and strength. Just as a gardener must understand the soil and climate to nourish their plants, so must you know your body and mind to cultivate a routine that truly nourishes you. Start by assessing your current physical condition, emotional state, and daily schedule. Are you dealing with chronic pain? Do you feel stressed or disconnected? How much time can you realistically dedicate to your practice each day? Answering these questions provides a foundation upon which you can build a personalized routine that not only addresses your specific needs but also fits seamlessly into your lifestyle.

For instance, if you find that stress is a constant in your life, incorporating exercises that focus on relaxation and breath control can be particularly beneficial. On the other hand, if you're recovering from an injury, your routine might focus more on gentle stretches and strengthening exercises that do not strain your body but help in rehabilitation. Remember, the goal here isn't to push your limits but to gently guide your body and mind to a better state of health. Choose exercises that you enjoy and feel comfortable with; this ensures that your somatic practice is something you look forward to each day, rather than a chore. As you grow more acquainted with various exercises, continue to adjust your choices based on what feels good and what doesn't, which will help in maintaining a routine that is both enjoyable and beneficial.

Personalizing Your Practice for Maximum Benefit

Imagine your somatic routine as a tailor-made outfit, designed to fit perfectly and highlight your best features. To personalize your practice, consider not only your physical and emotional needs but also your preferences. Do you prefer a morning routine to energize you for the day or a calming evening sequence to help you unwind? Do you enjoy the quiet introspection of yoga, or do you find vibrant energy in dance-based movements? By aligning your somatic practice with your personal preferences, you increase the likelihood of its integration into your daily life.

Moreover, setting personal goals can guide your practice. Whether it's improving flexibility, enhancing mental clarity, or building strength, having clear goals can motivate you to stick to your routine and make it more rewarding. For each goal, identify specific exercises that contribute to achieving it. For example, if enhancing flexibility is your aim, incorporating a daily series of dynamic stretches can be effective. By continually aligning your practice with your goals, you ensure that each session is purposeful and steers you closer to your desired outcomes.

Adjusting Your Routine as You Grow

As with any aspect of life, change is inevitable in your somatic practice. As you evolve, so too will your needs and goals. It's important to remain open to this evolution and to adjust your routine accordingly. This might mean swapping out certain exercises that no longer serve you or increasing the intensity of your routine to match your improved physical capabilities. For example, you might start with basic yoga poses, and as you gain flexibility and strength, you might incorporate more advanced poses or sequences.

Regularly reassess your routine to ensure it continues to meet your changing needs. This doesn't have to be a daunting task; a simple monthly or quarterly review can suffice. During these reviews, reflect on what's working and what isn't, and consider any new challenges or goals that have arisen. This ongoing adjustment not only keeps your routine aligned with your current state but also keeps it dynamic and interesting, which can be crucial in maintaining your motivation and engagement.

Feedback Loops for Continuous Improvement

The concept of feedback loops is essential in any growth-oriented process. In the context of somatic exercises, this means creating a system where you regularly receive feedback on your progress, reflect on it, and make necessary adjustments. This could be as simple as keeping a journal where you record your feelings and any physical sensations during and after each session. Over time, this journal can provide insightful patterns that highlight the most beneficial aspects of your practice and areas for adjustment.

Another way to create feedback loops is through regular check-ins with a coach or trainer, who can provide professional insights into your progress and offer suggestions for enhancement. Alternatively, if you prefer a more community-oriented approach, joining a group class or online forum where experiences and tips can be shared can also serve as a valuable source of feedback.

By actively engaging in these feedback loops, you ensure that your somatic practice remains a living, breathing part of your journey toward wellness. It adapts with you, celebrates your progress, and supports you through challenges, making it a true companion in your quest for a healthier, more balanced life.

7.6 Overcoming Common Obstacles in Somatic Practice

Navigating the path to a consistent somatic practice is not without its hurdles. You might encounter days when your body feels too stiff to move fluidly, or moments when your mind rebels against the calm you're trying to achieve. Recognizing and overcoming these hurdles is crucial, not just for the advancement of your practice, but for personal growth and understanding.

Identifying Personal Obstacles

The first step in overcoming obstacles in your somatic practice is to identify them clearly. These can vary widely—from physical limitations like pain or discomfort to emotional barriers such as lack of motivation or fear of inadequacy. Sometimes, the obstacles might be logistical, like finding time in a crowded schedule or adequate space in a small home. Start by keeping a practice journal. Note any feelings of resistance, physical pain, or distractions that occur during your sessions. Over time, patterns will emerge, helping you pinpoint the specific obstacles that are holding you back. This personal insight is invaluable as it transforms vague frustrations into actionable challenges.

Strategies for Overcoming Resistance

Once you've identified your obstacles, the next step is to strategize on how to overcome them. If time constraints are an issue, consider micro-practices—a few minutes of deep breathing or a quick series of stretches that can be integrated into your daily routine without overwhelming it. For physical limitations, adapt your practice to accommodate your body's needs. This might mean modifying poses or pacing to avoid discomfort while still engaging in the practice. If motivation is your barrier, set small, achievable goals that give you a sense of accomplishment and propel you forward. For example, commit to just five minutes of practice every morning and gradually increase the time as you settle into a routine. Remember, the goal is progress, not perfection.

Maintaining Motivation and Consistency

Keeping the flame of motivation alive requires nurturing. One effective method is to connect your practice to your deeper life values. Perhaps you value health because it allows you to be active with your kids, or maybe mental clarity enables you to perform at your best at work. Linking your somatic practice to these meaningful aspects of your life can provide the motivation to stick with it even when it's challenging. Additionally, consistency can be fostered by creating rituals around your practice. Maybe you light a candle before you begin, or play a particular piece of music that signals to your body and mind that it's time to engage in somatics. Over time, these rituals become signals that prepare you internally for the practice, making it easier to transition into the space of mindfulness and movement.

These strategies are designed not just to help you overcome obstacles but also to transform your practice into a more meaningful and sustainable part of your life. They encourage a deeper connection with your own needs and a more compassionate approach to your limitations and challenges. As you continue to navigate these hurdles, remember that each challenge overcome is a step towards deeper self-understanding and greater physical and emotional health.

In concluding this chapter on integrating practical tips into your daily somatic practice, we've explored a variety of strategies tailored to fit the realities of busy schedules, personal and professional goals, and nutritional support, all designed to enhance the effectiveness and enjoyment of your somatic journey. As we move forward, these foundational elements prepare us to delve deeper into advanced techniques and broaden our understanding of how somatic practices can continue to evolve and enrich our lives in the chapters to come.

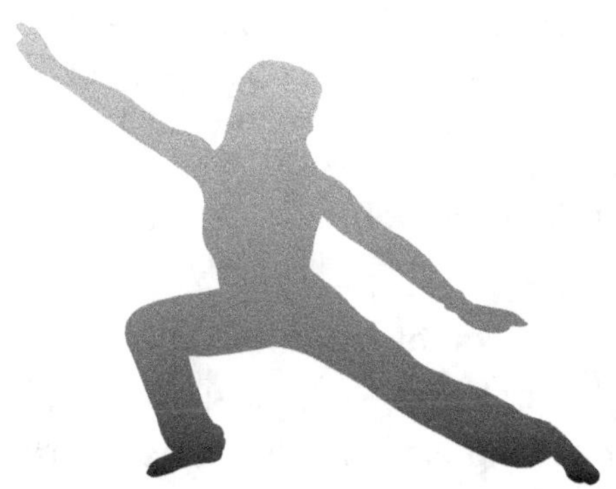

Chapter 8: Advanced Techniques and Continuing Your Journey

Imagine standing at a crossroads in a lush and expansive forest, where each path leads to new depths of discovery about your own capabilities and wellness. This chapter is your guide to choosing the path that deepens your connection to your body and mind through advanced somatic techniques. As you've grown more comfortable with the foundational practices, it's time to explore how intensified efforts and refined techniques can further enhance your journey. Here, we delve into advanced breathing techniques that promise not only to refine your somatic practice but to infuse your daily life with a renewed sense of vitality and harmony.

8.1 Deepening Your Practice: Advanced Breathing Techniques

Exploring Advanced Breathwork

Breathing, an act as natural as it is vital, holds the key to a profound depth of tranquility and power within you. As you advance in your somatic journey, exploring sophisticated breathwork techniques can unlock levels of body-mind integration that you might have only glimpsed in earlier stages. Techniques such as Pranayama in yoga offer an array of breathing practices, each with unique benefits. For instance, Kapalabhati (Skull Shining Breath) invigorates the body and clears the mind, while Nadi Shodhana (Alternate Nostril Breathing) balances the body's energy channels, harmonizing your emotional landscape. These practices deepen your breath's impact, enhancing oxygen flow and energy release, which catalyzes a more profound internal experience during each session.

Breathing Techniques for Advanced Practitioners

For those ready to deepen their practice, incorporating these advanced techniques can be transformative. Let's explore Bhastrika, or Bellows Breath, known for its energizing quality. This vigorous breathing technique involves a series of rapid, forceful inhales and exhales through the nose, akin to the bellows used to fuel a fire. It's designed to increase your Prana, or life energy, stimulating both physical and mental vitality. Practicing Bhastrika at the beginning of your day can awaken your senses and prepare you for the challenges ahead, infusing you with a robust energy that sustains you through your daily activities.

Integrating Advanced Breathwork into Daily Life

Integrating these powerful breathing techniques into your daily routine can enhance your well-being significantly. Imagine using Sitali, the Cooling Breath, to manage stress on a hectic day or to cool down physically and mentally after a strenuous activity. To practice Sitali, simply curl your tongue lengthwise and breathe in through it like a straw, then close your mouth and exhale through your nose. This technique is particularly effective in reducing emotional and physical heat, promoting a calm, cool demeanor that can transform your approach to stressful situations.

The Role of Breath in Advanced Somatic Practices

In advanced somatic practices, breath acts as a bridge between the physical and the subtle, the body and the mind. Each advanced technique you incorporate not only enhances your physical flexibility and strength but also deepens your mental focus and emotional resilience. The rhythmic cadence of controlled breathing can help synchronize your bodily functions, leading to enhanced harmony and efficiency in every breath, movement, and thought. As you continue to practice, you may find that these breathing techniques not only improve your somatic exercises but also imbue every moment of your day with a greater sense of peace and presence.

Interactive Element: Journaling Prompt

To truly harness the benefits of advanced breathwork, consider maintaining a breathwork journal. After each session, jot down the technique used, your emotional state before and after, and any physical sensations experienced during the practice. Over time, this journal can become a valuable tool for understanding the impact of each technique on your body and mind, helping you to fine-tune your practice to better meet your personal health and wellness goals.

As you continue to explore these advanced breathing techniques, remember that each breath is a step deeper into the sanctuary of your own body and mind. With each inhale and exhale, you're not only nourishing your body with oxygen but also nurturing a profound connection with the essence of your being. These practices are keys to unlocking the fullest potential of your breath and your ability to influence your health and well-being profoundly. By integrating these techniques into your daily routine, you ensure that your journey through somatic practices is not just maintained but also enriched, continuing to grow in depth and satisfaction.

8.2 Exploring the Bound Angle Pose for Advanced Practitioners

The Bound Angle Pose, known as Baddha Konasana in Sanskrit, offers a beautiful exploration into the depths of hip openness and the subtle layers of emotional release that this physical opening can initiate. *As you sit, the soles of your feet pressed together, knees falling gently to the sides, you are not merely performing a stretch; you are engaging in a dialogue with your body, listening to the whispers of tight muscles and perhaps, the echoes of stored emotions. This pose is revered not only for its ability to enhance flexibility and pelvic health but also for its profound impact on emotional well-being, making it a cornerstone in the practice of advanced yogis and anyone delving deeper into holistic health practices.*

Deepening Hip Openers

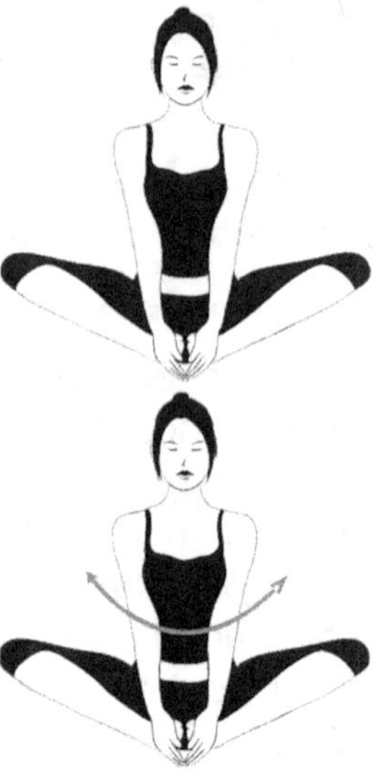

The hips are often termed the seat of our emotions, a place where stress, trauma, and daily pressures can unconsciously accumulate. The Bound Angle Pose acts as a key to unlocking these areas, offering a pathway to release and relief. To deepen your experience in this pose, focus on maintaining a tall, elongated spine, which enhances the stretch and prevents any rounding of the back that might shift the focus away from the hips. Gradually ease your knees closer to the floor, but be mindful of any discomfort; the goal is a gentle opening, not forcing the body beyond its limits. Over time, as your hips begin to open, you may find a decrease in back pain and an increase in your overall range of motion, benefits that extend well beyond the mat.

Techniques for Safely Advancing in the Pose

Advancing in the Bound Angle Pose requires more than physical flexibility; it demands patience and attentiveness to the body's subtle cues. Begin each session by warming up your body with gentler stretches such as the Easy Pose or the Pigeon Pose to prepare your hips and lower back. As you move into the Bound Angle Pose, use props like cushions or blocks under each knee to support your thighs, allowing you to maintain the pose longer without strain. Focus on breathing deeply, using each exhale to gently deepen the stretch. This mindful progression ensures that you enhance your flexibility while honoring your body's current boundaries, reducing the risk of injury.

Integrating the Pose into a Holistic Practice

Incorporating the Bound Angle Pose into your holistic somatic routine can amplify its benefits, making it a powerful tool for both physical and emotional health. Consider pairing this pose with breathwork that focuses on deep abdominal breathing to enhance relaxation and increase the emotional release. Following the pose with a few minutes of meditation can also help in assimilating the emotional shifts and physical sensations experienced during the practice. This integration creates a comprehensive routine that not only stretches the body but also soothes the mind and nurtures the spirit, embodying the essence of holistic health.

The Role of the Bound Angle Pose in Emotional Release

The process of releasing emotions through hip-opening poses like the Bound Angle Pose is both subtle and profound. As your physical body relaxes and opens, you may find that emotions you've been holding onto begin to surface. This is a natural part of the process and signifies a release of energy that has potentially been stored in the body for a long time. Embrace these moments with kindness and allow yourself to feel and release these emotions without judgment. This emotional cleansing can lead to a significant reduction in stress and anxiety, contributing to a more balanced and peaceful state of being. As you continue to practice, you might discover a deeper sense of emotional resilience and an enhanced capacity to handle life's stresses, making the Bound Angle Pose a valuable ally in your journey toward emotional and physical health.

Each session in the Bound Angle Pose offers a unique opportunity to connect deeply with your body and emotions, exploring the intricate dance between physical openness and emotional liberation. As you continue to engage with this pose, let it be a mirror reflecting not only your physical flexibility but also your emotional openness and depth, highlighting the profound interconnectedness of your body and mind.

8.3 The Role of Mindful Eating in Somatic Awareness

Imagine sitting down to a meal, seeing it not just as nourishment for your body, but as an integral part of your somatic practice, a true union of your physical and emotional self-care routines. Mindful eating and somatic awareness are deeply interconnected, each practice enhancing and supporting the other in a symbiotic relationship. Mindful eating involves paying full attention to the experience of eating and drinking, both inside and outside the body. It encourages you to notice the colors, smells, textures, flavors, temperatures, and even the sounds of your food. You're also invited to observe the responses your body has to your food—the signals of hunger and satiety, the connection to craving, and the feelings that associate with different foods.

This deep attention enhances your somatic awareness, making you more attuned to the needs and signals of your body—not just while eating, but in all aspects of life. For instance, as you become more aware of how certain foods affect your energy and mood, you might start to notice how other aspects of your environment affect your physical and emotional state. This heightened awareness can transform your approach to eating from a routine task to an intentional practice that supports your overall well-being.

Practices for Mindful Eating

Engaging in mindful eating is like tuning an instrument before a performance; it's about preparing your body and mind to engage fully and harmoniously with the task at hand. Start by serving yourself smaller portions to avoid automatic overeating. Before you begin eating, take a moment to appreciate the appearance and aroma of your food, which can help stimulate digestion.

As you eat, put down your utensils between bites, chew thoroughly, and try to identify all the ingredients, especially seasonings, in your dish. This not only slows down your eating pace but also increases your appreciation for the food. Additionally, try to eliminate distractions at meals—turn off the TV, put away your phone, and avoid reading. This helps you focus on the eating experience, making it easier to listen to your body's signals of fullness and satisfaction.

Integrating these practices into your daily routine might seem challenging at first, especially if you're used to eating on the go or while multitasking. However, the benefits of this practice are profound, extending beyond just better digestion and weight management. Mindful eating helps reduce binge eating and emotional eating behaviors by improving your response to emotional cues—instead of eating automatically in response to stress or boredom, you learn to pause, assess your actual needs, and respond appropriately.

Integrating Mindful Eating into Your Somatic Practice

To weave mindful eating into your somatic practice, consider starting or ending your exercise routine with a mindful eating exercise. For example, you might begin a yoga session by mindfully eating a small piece of fruit, focusing fully on the experience. This sets a tone of mindfulness and presence that carries through into your physical practice. Alternatively, conclude a session with a mindful meal or snack, using the calm and centered state induced by your workout to truly savor and digest your food.

This integration encourages a holistic approach to well-being, where mindfulness permeates all aspects of your life, enhancing both your physical health and your emotional resilience. As you continue to practice both mindful eating and somatic exercises, you may find that each enhances the sensitivity and awareness cultivated by the other, leading to greater body-mind integration and overall health.

Nutrition's Impact on Somatic Sensitivity

The foods you choose to eat can significantly affect your somatic sensitivity, either dampening or enhancing your body's signals. For example, foods high in sugar and artificial additives may cloud your body's natural cues, leading to overstimulation or a numbing of body awareness. Conversely, a diet rich in whole foods, such as vegetables, fruits, whole grains, and lean proteins, can enhance your sensitivity to your body's needs. These foods provide a steady supply of energy and nutrients, without the dramatic blood sugar spikes and crashes that can obscure somatic awareness.

Incorporating anti-inflammatory foods like turmeric, ginger, and fatty fish can also enhance somatic sensitivity by reducing chronic inflammation, which may otherwise mask subtle cues from your body. Similarly, incorporating foods rich in magnesium, such as leafy greens and nuts, can help relax your muscles and nervous system, enhancing your ability to tune into your body during somatic practices.

As you explore the deep connections between what you eat and how you feel, both physically and emotionally, mindful eating can become not just a practice but a way of life. This approach not only enhances your somatic practices but also enriches your overall experience of health and vitality, making every meal a step towards greater self-awareness and well-being.

8.4 Somatic Exercises for Specific Conditions: Tailoring Your Practice

When you think of somatic exercises, it's easy to envision a one-size-fits-all approach, but the truth is far more personal and profound. Each of us carries unique stories in our bodies—histories of pain, joy, trauma, and healing. These narratives deeply influence how we move and exist in our spaces. Recognizing and honoring this individuality is crucial, especially when adapting somatic exercises to cater to specific health conditions or injuries. This sensitivity not only ensures safety but also maximizes the effectiveness of each movement, making your practice a true ally in your health journey.

Customizing Your Practice for Health Conditions

Tailoring somatic exercises to address specific health conditions begins with an understanding of the condition itself and its impact on your body. This might mean consulting with healthcare providers to understand the dos and don'ts specific to your situation. For instance, if you are managing a condition like arthritis, your focus might be on exercises that enhance joint mobility and reduce stiffness without causing pain. Techniques such as gentle joint rotations or soft stretches that emphasize fluidity over force can be particularly beneficial. Similarly, for those recovering from cardiac issues, exercises that gently elevate the heart rate and improve circulation, like slow-paced walking or light yoga, may be recommended. It's about finding what enriches your body's capability without pushing it into discomfort, thus fostering a healing environment.

Somatic Practices for Pain Management

Pain management is another area where somatic exercises excel, offering relief and rehabilitation in ways that are both gentle and profound. The key here is to focus on exercises that not only alleviate pain but also address its underlying causes. For instance, chronic back pain can often be mitigated through exercises that strengthen the core, supporting the spine, and thus reducing strain. Practices like pelvic tilts or gentle supine twists can be incredibly effective. Additionally, incorporating mindfulness and breathwork into these exercises can enhance their pain-relieving effects. By focusing deeply on the breath and the body's responses during each movement, you can help interrupt the cycle of chronic pain, offering not just momentary relief but a potential long-term solution.

Adapting Somatic Exercises for Different Abilities

Ensuring that somatic exercises are inclusive and accessible is fundamental. This might mean adapting exercises to be performed while seated or using props like chairs or cushions for support. For example, a chair can be used to modify yoga poses, making them accessible to those who cannot perform floor-based exercises. Similarly, for individuals with limited mobility, exercises can be adapted to focus on the upper body or even just on breathing and relaxation techniques. The aim is to make somatic practices a welcoming space for everyone, regardless of physical capability, ensuring that each person can engage in a way that feels supportive and enriching.

Guidance for Safe Practice

Navigating the landscape of somatic exercises safely requires an awareness of your body's cues and sometimes, the guidance of professionals. It's crucial to listen to your body and avoid pushing into pain. Pain is a clear signal from your body to stop and reassess. Moreover, if you're dealing with a specific health condition or recovering from an injury, professional guidance can be invaluable. A physical therapist or a certified somatic exercise coach can tailor your practice to your specific needs, ensuring safety and effectiveness. They can also help you progress at a pace that supports your healing, helping you find the balance between challenge and care.

In your personal practice, always start with a warm-up to prepare your body for exercise and end with a cool-down to return to a resting state gently. These practices reduce the risk of injury and help integrate the benefits of the exercises into your body. Remember, the goal of adapting somatic exercises is not just to perform them but to integrate them into your life in a way that supports and enhances your health and well-being. As you continue to tailor these practices to your needs, you'll find that they not only improve your physical health but also enrich your connection with your body, empowering you to live more fully and comfortably.

8.5 Incorporating Somatics into Holistic Wellness Routines

Holistic wellness transcends the mere absence of disease—it's a vibrant state of health and vitality, achieved by living in balance and harmony with the mind, body, and spirit. Somatic practices play a crucial role in this holistic approach, providing tools to connect deeply with the body and manage stress effectively. These practices, which range from gentle stretches to focused breathing, encourage a mindfulness that helps bridge the gap between physical health and emotional resilience. Integrating somatic practices into your daily routine isn't just about adding more activities to your day—it's about enriching your life's tapestry, weaving in patterns that enhance your well-being at every level.

Combining Somatics with Other Wellness Modalities

Imagine your wellness routine as a symphony, each element contributing to a harmonious whole. Somatic practices, with their focus on bodily awareness and relaxation, blend beautifully with other wellness modalities such as meditation, yoga, and mindfulness. For instance, starting your morning with yoga can loosen and prepare your body, making subsequent meditation or mindfulness practices more profound and effective. During yoga, the physical poses help release bodily tensions that often hold emotional stress, clearing the way for deeper meditative states. Similarly, ending a session of vigorous somatic exercises with a few minutes of mindfulness can help consolidate the gains of your physical practice, allowing your body to integrate the changes and heal.

Creating a Balanced Wellness Routine

Achieving balance in your wellness routine means ensuring that each aspect of your health—physical, mental, and spiritual—is nurtured. This balance can be achieved by strategically scheduling different practices throughout your week. For example, you might dedicate mornings to somatic exercises that energize the body and prepare the mind for the day ahead. Evenings could be reserved for practices that calm and center, such as meditation or gentle yoga, helping to unwind the mind and ease the body into restorative sleep. It's also valuable to incorporate regular periods of reflection—perhaps through journaling or discussion with a wellness coach—to assess the effectiveness of your routine and make adjustments as needed. This ongoing evaluation ensures that your wellness routine remains responsive to your evolving needs and goals.

Evolving Your Wellness Routine with Somatics

As you grow in your somatic practice, you might find that your body and mind begin to crave deeper or more varied forms of engagement. This is a natural part of the growth process and a sign that your routine is due for an evolution. Introducing advanced somatic techniques or new modalities can reinvigorate your practice and challenge you in new ways. For instance, if you've been practicing basic body scans, you might progress to more nuanced forms of interoceptive awareness techniques, which can deepen your understanding of the body's internal signals. Alternatively, incorporating elements of dance therapy or advanced tai chi can provide new physical challenges while also enhancing emotional expression. This evolution in your practice keeps it dynamic and closely aligned with your personal growth, ensuring that it continues to support your holistic health effectively.

Incorporating somatic practices into your holistic wellness routine offers a pathway to deeper self-awareness and health. It requires a commitment not just to practicing regularly but to listening deeply to your body's needs and responding with care. Whether you are stretching, breathing, or simply sitting in mindful awareness, each practice is a step towards a more balanced and harmonious life. As you continue to weave these practices into your daily routine, they become less like tasks and more like parts of a beautiful dance, enhancing every aspect of your well-being and allowing you to move through life with greater ease and joy.

8.6 Next Steps: Continuing Your Somatic Journey Beyond the Basics

The path of somatic practices is not just about reaching a destination; it's about embracing a process of continuous growth and learning. As you deepen your engagement with somatic exercises, you'll find that the journey evolves, offering new landscapes of understanding and opportunities to refine your practices. Lifelong learning in the realm of somatics is pivotal—it keeps your practice vibrant and ensures that it continues to meet your changing needs and aspirations. This ongoing engagement with new techniques and insights not only enriches your personal practice but also keeps you connected to the evolving field of somatic health, which is continually enhanced by new research and methodologies.

Lifelong Learning and Somatic Practices

Think of your somatic practice as a garden that requires regular tending, not just for maintenance but for growth. Expanding your knowledge and skills is akin to introducing new plants to your garden—it enriches the ecosystem and increases its vibrancy. Engaging with advanced workshops, reading the latest books on body-mind integration, or even taking online courses can introduce you to new concepts and techniques that can be transformative for your practice. For example, learning about the latest research on neuroplasticity might inspire you to incorporate exercises that enhance brain function and emotional resilience. This commitment to ongoing education ensures that your practice remains dynamic and tailored to the latest understandings of body-mind health.

Finding Advanced Resources and Communities

As you seek to deepen your somatic knowledge, finding communities and resources that support your growth is essential. Look for workshops led by respected practitioners or join online forums where professionals and enthusiasts share insights and experiences. These communities can be invaluable sources of support and inspiration, offering perspectives that challenge and refine your own understanding of somatic practices. Additionally, attending conferences or joining professional associations related to somatics can keep you at the forefront of the field, ensuring that you are always connected to the latest developments and innovations.

Setting Long-Term Goals for Your Practice

To maintain direction and purpose in your practice, setting long-term goals is crucial. These goals should reflect both your personal aspirations and the broader possibilities of your somatic journey. Perhaps you aim to achieve a certain level of mastery in a specific technique or wish to explore how somatics can enhance other areas of your life, like creativity or spiritual development. By setting clear, achievable goals, you create a roadmap for your practice that not only guides your daily activities but also inspires continued growth and exploration.

Embracing the Evolving Nature of Somatic Work

Somatic practices are inherently dynamic, reflecting the continual changes in our bodies and lives. Embracing this evolving nature requires an openness to change and an understanding that your practices will need to adapt over time. This might mean modifying your routines as your body ages or as you encounter new health challenges. It also involves being open to new scientific discoveries that could alter your understanding of body-mind interactions. By staying flexible and responsive to change, you ensure that your somatic practice remains relevant and effective, providing you with the tools you need to manage your well-being in an ever-changing world.

In this chapter, we've explored how you can continue to grow and refine your somatic practice beyond the basics. By engaging in lifelong learning, connecting with communities, setting long-term goals, and embracing the evolving nature of somatic work, you ensure that your practice not only sustains you but also inspires and transforms you. As we move forward, remember that each step in this journey offers valuable opportunities for development and discovery, inviting you to explore the rich landscape of somatic practices with curiosity and enthusiasm.

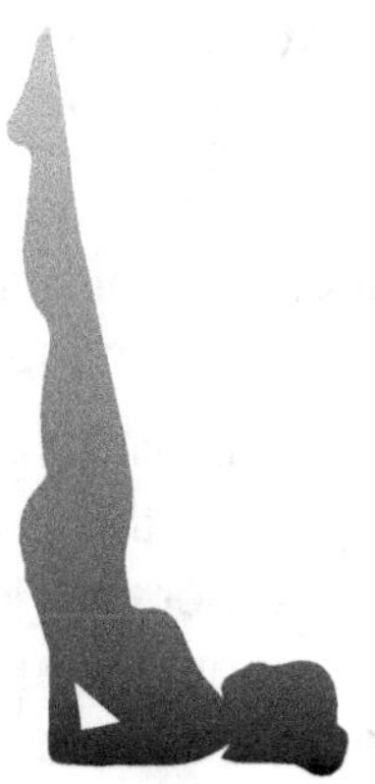

Conclusion

As we draw this journey through the pages of somatic practices to a close, I want to take a moment to reflect on the transformative passage we've navigated together. From the gentle stretches that unwind tension along your spine to the deep, rhythmic breathing that calms your bustling nerves, we've explored a variety of practices that not only reset your nervous system but also elevate your emotional awareness and resilience. This book has been a testament to the power of integrating body and mind through movements and mindfulness, each technique a step towards a more harmonious self.

Holistic wellness is not just a goal but a continuous journey that involves the integration of mind, body, and spirit. By combining somatic exercises with mindful breathing, nutritious eating, and other mindfulness practices, we have unlocked a comprehensive pathway to health. This approach isn't just about alleviating physical discomfort or fleeting stress - it's about cultivating a deep, enduring state of wellness that nourishes every part of your being.

One of the most beautiful aspects of somatic practices is their universality. Regardless of age, physical condition, or previous experience with holistic practices, these methods are accessible and adaptable. They are a testament to the inclusivity of wellness - a tool that belongs to everyone and can be tailored to fit each unique journey.

Throughout this book, we've delved into key techniques such as spine stretches, full body stretches, pelvic tilts, and vagus nerve stimulation. Each of these practices plays a vital role in enhancing your posture, increasing your flexibility, balancing your emotions, and ultimately, contributing to your overall happiness. The benefits are immense and, more importantly, achievable if integrated into your daily life. That's why I've emphasized the importance of weaving somatic exercises into your everyday routines, allowing the benefits to unfold gradually but significantly over time.

Acknowledging that the path to wellness is a continuous one, I encourage you to view this book not as a conclusion but as a beginning or a deepening of your journey. Each page turned, each practice tried, and each breath taken is a step forward in a much larger, ongoing journey of discovery and growth.

Now, let me extend a heartfelt call to action: Start today, no matter how small the step might seem. Embrace the practices discussed and trust in their potential to transform. Remember, the journey to wellness begins with a single, mindful step. Start where you are, use what you have, and do what you can. Your body and mind will thank you.

I am deeply grateful for your companionship on this journey. Remember that you are not alone as you continue to explore and expand your somatic practices. The road to wellness is often shared, and there is a vibrant community of practitioners and learners who are on this path with you. Engage with them, share your experiences, and support each other in this beautiful pursuit of health and happiness.

If you find yourself facing obstacles or setbacks, remember that these are natural parts of any journey. Persistence, patience, and consistency in your practice will guide you through these challenges and lead to profound personal growth and healing.

Finally, let me leave you with this thought: You have within you the power to cultivate a life of balance and harmony. Each breath, each stretch, and each moment of mindfulness adds a thread to the tapestry of your well-being. Continue to weave this tapestry with intention and joy, knowing that each day brings new opportunities for health and happiness.

Thank you for allowing me to guide you through these practices. May your path be filled with learning, health, and tranquility. Remember, the journey is as beautiful as the destination, and you have everything you need to make it a wonderful one.

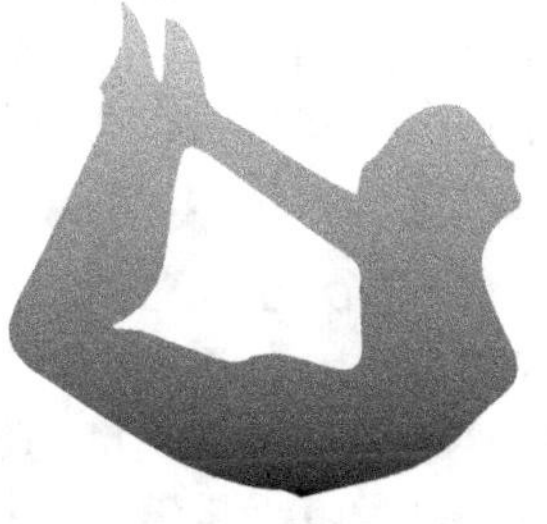

References

- *Somatic Movement: What It Is, Benefits, and Tips - Peloton* https://www.onepeloton.com/blog/somatic-movement/

- Zaccaro, A., Piarulli, A., Laurino, M., Garbella, E., Menicucci, D., Neri, B., & Gemignani, A. (2018). *How Breath-Control Can Change Your Life: A Systematic Review on Psycho-Physiological Correlates of Slow Breathing* (Vol. 12). PubMed. https://doi.org/10.3389/fnhum.2018.00353

- Howland, R. H. (2014). Vagus nerve stimulation. *Current Behavioral Neuroscience Reports*, *1*(2), 64–73. https://doi.org/10.1007/s40473-014-0010-5

- *Integrating Mindfulness and Somatic Therapy for Cultural Healing* https://byrepose.com/journal/integrating-mindfulness-and-somatic-therapy-for-cultural-healing

- Silva, L. (2024). What is somatic therapy? Benefits, types and efficacy. *Forbes Health*. https://www.forbes.com/health/mind/somatic-therapy/#:~:text=Somatic%20therapy%20may%20increase%20an,%2Dbeing%2C%20according%20to%20research.

- DiNardo, K. (2018, August 24). *Create your own meditation space.* AARP. Retrieved April 29, 2024, from https://www.aarp.org/home-family/your-home/info-2018/create-meditation-space.html

- Dernovsek, S. (2019, October 29). *What is the somatic approach to yoga?* YogaAnytime. Retrieved April 29, 2024, from https://www.yogaanytime.com/blog/asana/what-is-the-somatic-approach-to-yoga

- *Integrating Somatic Practices into Everyday Life — Repose* https://byrepose.com/journal/integrating-somatic-practices-into-everyday-life

- Bachert, A. (2024, January 17). *Try these somatic exercises to improve your mental health*. CharlieHealth. Retrieved April 29, 2024, from https://www.charliehealth.com/post/somatic-exercises-for-mental-health

- Mayo clinc. (2020). Pelvic tilt exercise. *Mayo Clinic*. https://www.mayoclinic.org/healthy-lifestyle/labor-and-delivery/multimedia/pelvic-tilt-exercise/img-20006410#:~:text=Do%20the%20pelvic%20tilt%20to,for%20up%20to%2010%20seconds.

- Nevaeh, M. (2024, April 2). *Yoga and mindfulness: elevating your practice through meditation and breathwork*. Medium. Retrieved April 29, 2024, from https://medium.com/@monaynevaeh/yoga-and-mindfulness-elevating-your-practice-through-meditation-and-breathwork-e605735a2b93

- Meehan, E., & Carter, B. (2021). Moving with Pain: What principles from somatic practices can offer to people living with chronic pain. *Frontiers in Psychology, 11*. https://doi.org/10.3389/fpsyg.2020.620381

- Knight, J. (2021, March 13). *3 Somatic movement yoga flows to promote better posture*. YogaU. Retrieved April 29, 2024, from https://yogauonline.com/yoga-health-benefits/posture-improvement/3-somatic-movement-yoga-flows-to-promote-better-posture/

- *Integrating Breathwork for Mindful Somatic Therapy Practice* https://healflow.org/integrating-breathwork-for-mindful-somatic-therapy-practice/

- Wong, A. (2023, August 27). *Reset your nervous System: Somatic tools for vagal tone*. Somatopia. Retrieved April 29, 2024, from https://www.somatopia.com/blog/reset-your-nervous-system-somatic-tools-for-vagal-tone

- Bach, D., Groesbeck, G., Stapleton, P., Sims, R., Blickheuser, K., & Church, D. (2019). Clinical EFT (Emotional Freedom Techniques) improves multiple physiological markers of health. *Journal of Evidence-based Integrative Medicine, 24*, 2515690X1882369. https://doi.org/10.1177/2515690x18823691

- Coates, H. (2024). How vagus nerve stimulation can help lower your stress levels. *Glamour*. https://www.glamour.com/story/how-vagus-nerve-stimulation-can-help-lower-your-stress-levels#:~:text=%E2%80%9CIt's%20like%20going%20to%20the,%2C%20recharge%2C%20and%20recover.%E2%80%9D

- Sutton, J. (2020, July 15). *Mindful Walking & Walking Meditation: a restorative practice*. Positive Psychology. Retrieved April 29, 2024, from https://positivepsychology.com/mindful-walking/

- Scott, E. (2024). What is body scan meditation? *VeryWellMind*. https://www.verywellmind.com/body-scan-meditation-why-and-how-3144782

- Meehan, E., & Carter, B. (2021b). Moving with Pain: What principles from somatic practices can offer to people living with chronic pain. *Frontiers in Psychology, 11*. https://doi.org/10.3389/fpsyg.2020.620381

- *Somatic Yoga Exercises, enhance your body awareness*. (2024, March 14). Dr Tara Salay. Retrieved April 29, 2024, from https://drtarasalay.com/somatic-yoga-exercises/

- Beck, K., Thomson, J. S., Swift, R. J., & Von Hurst, P. (2015). Role of nutrition in performance enhancement and postexercise recovery. *Open Access Journal of Sports Medicine*, 259. https://doi.org/10.2147/oajsm.s33605

- Blanton, K. (2024). Somatic Exercises: how it works, stretching, and moves for beginners. *Prevention*. https://www.prevention.com/fitness/workouts/a46993501/somatic-exercises/?utm_source=google&utm_medium=cpc&utm_campaign=arb_ga_pre_md_pmx_hybd_mix_ca_20739843272&gad_source=1&gclid=Cj0KCQjwir2xBhC_ARIsAMTXk87sakSsffQNqP6C4RyOg6Bqq-40v93nytQAMBV9uqVRjlvATzCeKflaAte-EALw_wcB

- Mateus, C. (2024, April 8). *Exploring the benefits: How somatic exercises can aid in weight loss*. Juniper. Retrieved April 29, 2024, from https://www.myjuniper.com/blog/somatic-exercises-for-weight-loss

- Stevens, C. (2023, November 24). *Constructive rest pose for Total-Body relaxation*. Livestrong. Retrieved April 29, 2024, from https://www.livestrong.com/article/13778605-constructive-rest-pose/

- Duvall, S. E. (2019, July 29). *Top 5 Pelvic Floor Exercises*. CoreExerciseSolutions. https://www.coreexercisesolutions.com/articles/best-pelvic-floor-exercises/*Try These Somatic Exercises to Improve Your Mental Health* https://www.charliehealth.com/post/somatic-exercises-for-mental-health

- *Mindful Walking: Stay Grounded by Walking Mindfully*. (n.d.). Mindfulness. Retrieved April 29, 2024, from https://mindfulness.com/mindful-living/mindful-walking

- Fowler, P. (2024). Breathing techniques for stress relief. *WebMD*. https://www.webmd.com/balance/stress-management/stress-relief-breathing-techniques

- Juntwait, K. (2023, May 16). *Your intro guide to starting a somatic exercise program*. TheWorkoutWitch. Retrieved April 29, 2024, from https://theworkoutwitch.com/en-ca/blogs/news/somatic-exercise-101-your-intro-guide-to-starting-a-somatic-exercise-program

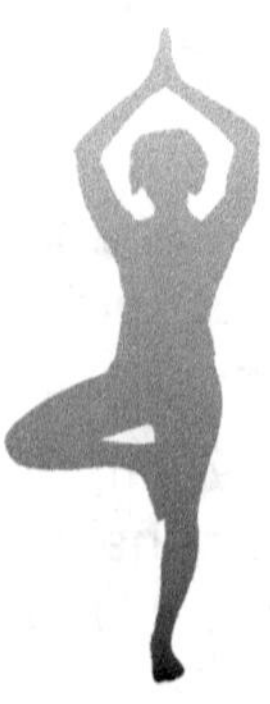

Cat-Cow Stretch

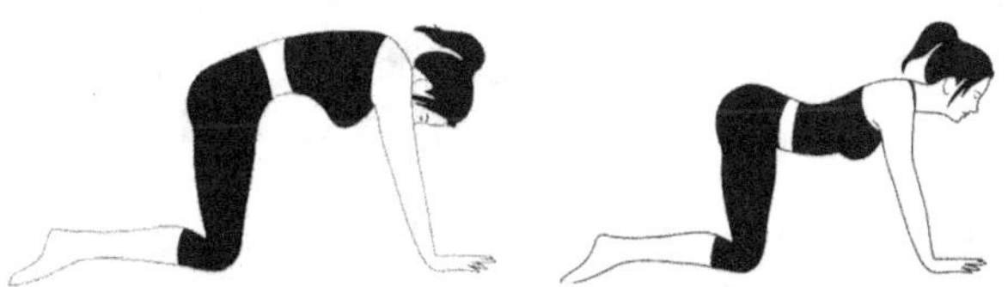

Positioning yourself on your hands and knees and gently alternating between arching your back towards the ceiling and dipping it towards the floor.

Gentle Full Body Stretch

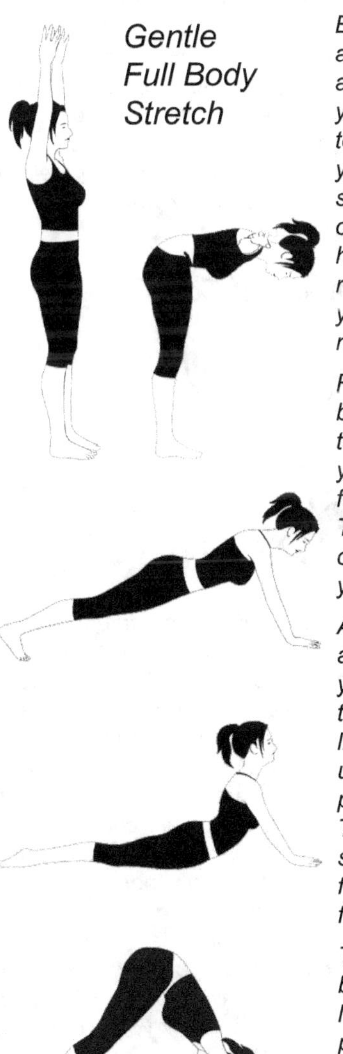

Begin with your feet hip-width apart, standing tall, and take a deep, grounding breath. As you exhale, reach your arms towards the sky, lengthening your entire body. After a few seconds, gently swan dive over your legs, letting your head hang and your neck relax, feeling the stretch in your hamstrings and the release in your lower back.

From this forward fold, step back into a plank position, taking a moment to ensure your body is in a straight line from your head to your heels. This not only engages your core but also strengthens your shoulders and arms.

After holding the plank for a few breaths, slowly lower your body to the ground and transition into a cobra pose by lifting your chest off the floor, using your back muscles to pull your torso back and up. This opens up your chest and shoulders, counteracting the forward hunch that comes from sitting at a desk.

To complete the cycle, push back into a downward dog, lifting your hips high and pressing your heels towards the ground, feeling the stretch in your calves and the decompression in your spine.

Spinal Twist

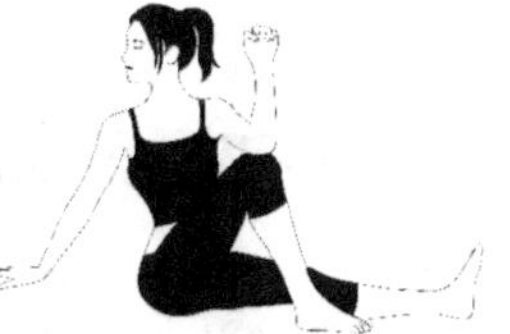

Sitting on the floor with your legs extended, bend one knee and place the opposite elbow on the outside of the bent knee, gently twisting your torso and looking over your shoulder.

'Wrist Walk' up a wall

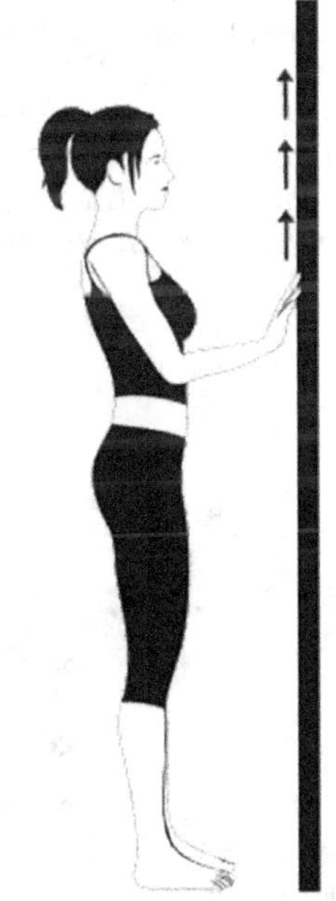

Face a wall, placing your palms against it at waist height, and slowly walking your fingers upwards, stretching the arms fully, then walking them back down. This not only stretches the elbow joints but also engages the muscles of the arms and shoulders, promoting blood flow and flexibility.

Superman Pose

Performing the Superman pose starts with you lying face down on a comfortable surface, arms extended in front of you, and legs stretched out behind. As you lift your arms and legs simultaneously, aiming to raise them a few inches off the ground, you engage not just the lower back but the entire lineup of muscles running along your spine and core. Hold this lifted position for a few seconds, feeling the gentle pull along your back and the engagement of your abdominal muscles. It's crucial to keep your head and neck in a neutral position, aligned with your spine, to avoid any strain. Exhale as you gently lower your limbs back to the starting position, and allow yourself a moment to relax before repeating the movement.

Wall Butterfly Pose

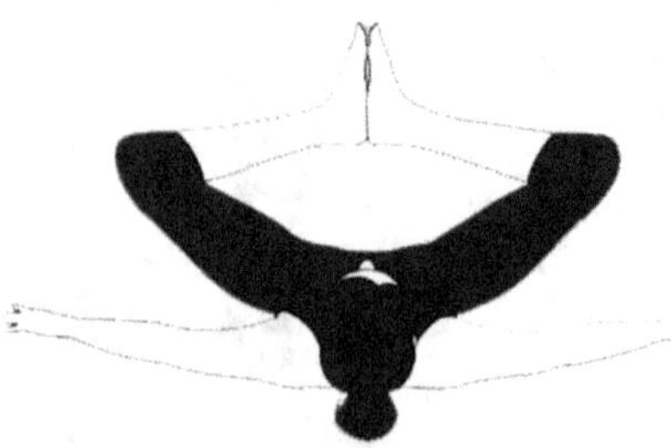

Start by sitting with your back straight against a wall, which provides support and alignment for your spine. Bring the soles of your feet together in front of you, drawing them as close to your body as feels comfortable. The closer your feet are to your body, the deeper the stretch, but it's important to proceed gradually and listen to your body's cues. Let your knees fall gently to the sides, feeling the stretch in your inner thighs and hips. The contact with the wall helps keep your spine from rounding, which is crucial for protecting your back during this stretch.

Seated Straddle Pose

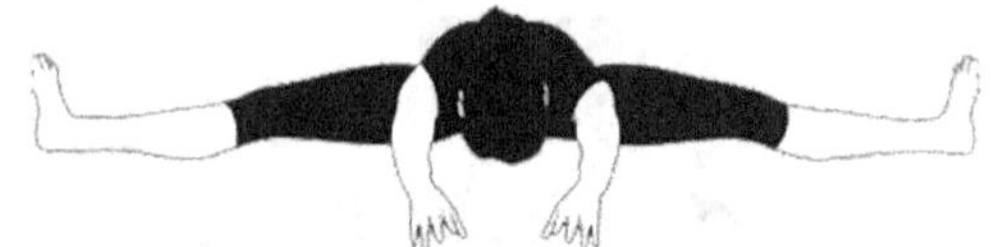

Start by sitting with your legs as wide apart as comfortably possible and your toes pointing upwards. Keep your spine straight and tall, imagining a string pulling you up from the top of your head. This alignment is crucial as it prevents unnecessary strain on your back. Lean forward from the hips, not the waist, to keep the spine elongated rather than curved. This forward motion should be guided by your breath: inhale to prepare, and exhale as you ease deeper into the stretch. Your hands can rest gently on the floor in front of you, helping to support your upper body and control the intensity of the stretch.

Seated Cat Cow Pose

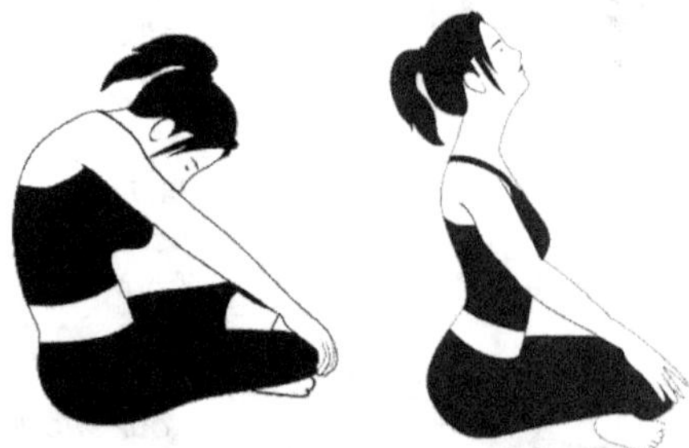

Start by finding a comfortable seated position on the floor or on a chair with your feet flat on the ground. If you're on the floor, cross your legs comfortably, ensuring your spine is straight and your shoulders are relaxed. Place your hands on your knees, which will help in facilitating the movement. As you inhale, arch your back slightly, pushing your chest forward and upward, and tilt your head back, opening your throat. This is the 'Cow' position, where you expose your heart and belly, inviting openness and vulnerability. As you transition into the 'Cat' position on your exhale, round your spine outward, draw your belly in, drop your head forward, and allow your shoulders to curve forward. This movement is about releasing and letting go, just as much as it is about engaging and strengthening.

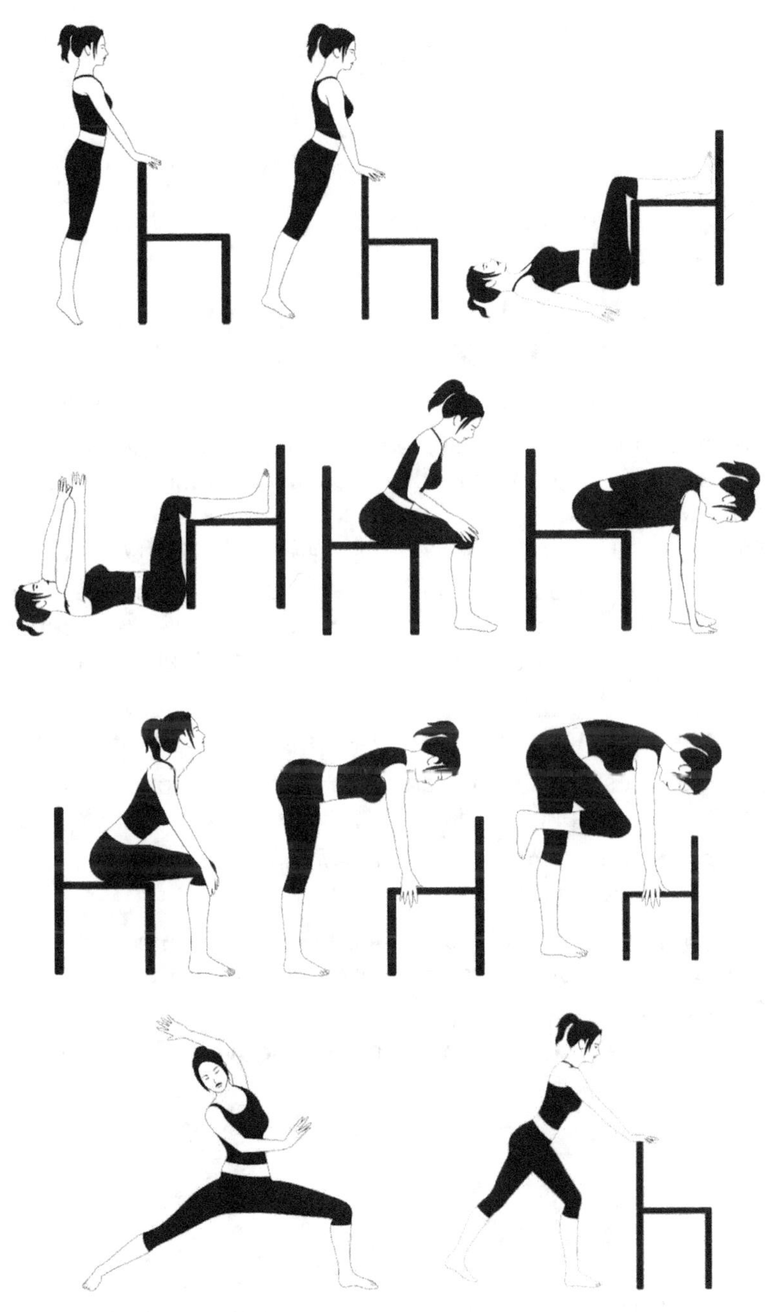

Bonus Exercises

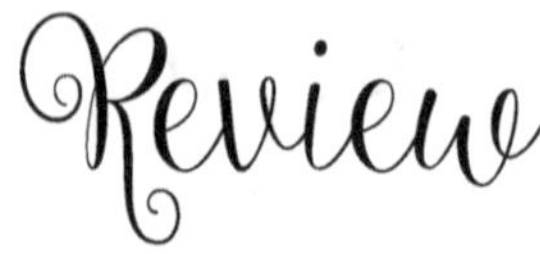

Review

Make a Difference with Your Review
Unlock the Power of Generosity

"The best way to find yourself is to lose yourself in the service of others."

Mahatma Gandhi

My mission is to help every woman unlock their inner strength and vitality through Somatic Exercises for All Women. Everything I do stems from that mission. And, the only way for me to accomplish that mission is by reaching… well….everyone.

This is where you come in. Most people do, in fact, judge a book by its cover (and its reviews). So here's my ask on behalf of every woman who is seeking to enhance their health and happiness:

Please help those women by leaving this book a Review.

Your gift costs no money and less than 60 seconds to make real, but it can change a fellow Empowered Woman's life forever.

Your review could help...one more woman transform her life……one more dream come true.

To get that 'feel good' feeling and help these women for real, all you have to do is... and it takes less than 60 seconds... Leave a Review.

Simply scan the QR code below to leave your review:

If you feel good about helping a fellow Empowered Woman, you are my kind of person. Welcome to the Club. You are one of us.

Your biggest fan,

L. R. Lepage,

Body Talk Practitioner and Author